An Examiner's Guide to Professional Plastic Surgery Exams

Michael F. Klaassen • Earle Brown

An Examiner's Guide to Professional Plastic Surgery Exams

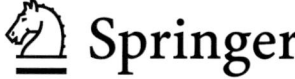 Springer

Michael F. Klaassen
Private Practice
Auckland
New Zealand

Earle Brown
Former Head of Department
Plastic Surgery Unit
Middlemore Hospital
Auckland
New Zealand

ISBN 978-981-13-0688-4   ISBN 978-981-13-0689-1   (eBook)
https://doi.org/10.1007/978-981-13-0689-1

Library of Congress Control Number: 2018948187

This Springer imprint is published by Springer Nature, under the registered company Springer Nature Singapore Pte Ltd.
The registered company address is: 152 Beach Road, #21-01/04 Gateway East, Singapore 189721, Singapore

Overview

Experience in both examining and preparing candidates for the Royal Australasian College of Surgeons final fellowship exam in plastic and reconstructive surgery over more than 15 years has been the impetus for this book. The FRACS exam is a gruelling experience for trainee plastic surgeons who have completed 5 years of advanced training in New Zealand and Australia. The reality is that the intense clinical workload in accredited service hospitals, may not always align with the topics that will be presented to them in the formal exam environment.

After 8 years of running an annual coaching course to help candidates prepare for the exams shortly before they begin, several important principles have emerged. Knowledge, judgement, decision-making and communicative interaction with the examiners and the clinical cases presented to them are some of the key strategies. Coping with the pressure, balancing all the performance aspects and learning to perform in the right exam environment are just some of the required skill set. This will be explored by a team of clinicians experienced in many different aspects of plastic surgery, anaesthesia and clinical psychology.

This book is the A–Z for trainees preparing for the final fellowship exam at least a year away. It discusses the basics (how to stay healthy and fresh in mind) as well as the specific details of writing exam answers, coping with the stress of oral exams and performing with your best face and brain, dealing with disappointment and how to begin your professional career once you succeed. Quintessentially it focuses on principles and maxims that have been shared with us by the giants of plastic surgery over the centuries … on whose shoulders we sit.

It is a book that is based on decades of surgical experience and our own experiences of being examined and examining. Both sides of the table are considered, and current examiners may wish to consider it as well.

Auckland, New Zealand   Michael F. Klaassen, FRACS
Auckland, New Zealand   Earle Brown, FRCS, FRACS
July 2018

Foreword

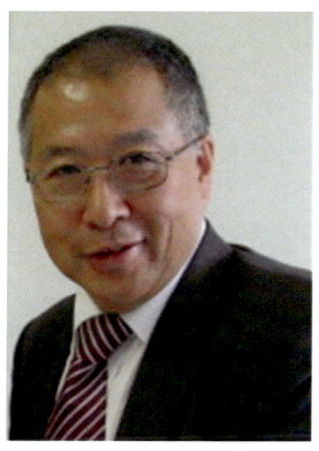

Considering the depth and scope of plastic and reconstructive surgery required in the Australasian (NZ and Australia) Fellowship Examination, this is probably one of the most difficult examinations to pass.

This book by Drs Klaassen and Brown gives an excellent analysis of each part of the examination. The first three chapters deal with the desired attitudes and psychology of sitting an examination.

The fourth chapter is on principles of plastic surgery. These are the words from the 'giants' in the field and are especially important, when the exam candidate faces an unusual and difficult clinical case.

The chapters thereafter detail each part of the examination, and they give the first-timer a realistic picture of the process.

Finally, with my previous experience as a senior examiner in plastic surgery, I find the Australasian Fellowship Examination to be a fair process, but it does require a deep knowledge, the right mental attitude and a good understanding of the examination process to be successful.

This book will assist the candidate in the last two requirements to pass the examination and would be beneficial to both the local trainees and international medical graduates.

Michael Leung, FRACS
Department of Plastic and Reconstructive Surgery
Monash Health
Melbourne, VIC, Australia

Preface

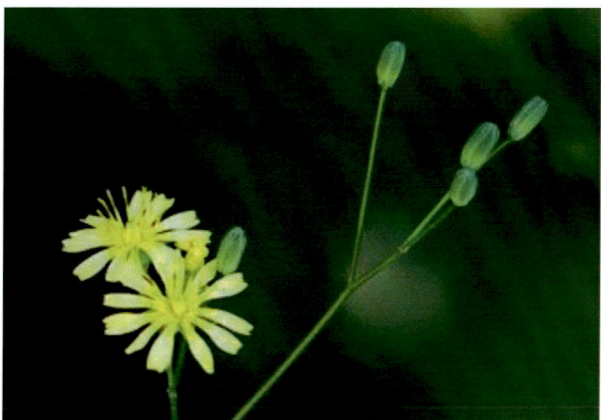

Lapsana Communis

Blackbird singing in the dead of the night
Take these broken wings and learn to fly
All your life
You were only waiting for this moment to arise

(Sir Paul McCartney)

The professional exams set by colleges, boards and institutions of plastic surgery are necessarily rigorous and demanding of a very high standard of competence.

This can be somewhat daunting for the examinee and equally challenging for the examiners. A sound knowledge of plastic surgery principles, philosophies, history and clinical management is required by the examinee to convince the examining court that they are ready—ready to step up to the role of a consultant plastic surgeon and all the responsibility that this implies.

Knowledge is not enough. Additional cognitive skills include comprehension, application, analysis, synthesis and evaluation: the ability to define, explain, interpret, distinguish, plan and judge any clinical situation in the clinic, in the operating room and on the ward round.

The Royal Australasian College of Surgeons (RACS), of which I became a fellow after many years of training and examination, defines nine competencies for the surgical trainee: teacher, scholar, health advocate, collaborator, medical expert, technical expert, communicator, leader, decision-maker and ethical practitioner.

After performing as an examiner for 8 years and then coaching candidates for another eight consecutive years, supported and encouraged by Dr Earle Brown, my mentor, I believe there are candidates for whom the exam can be a very unfair and stressful test. This was evident recently when a very competent and well-prepared candidate, with excellent prospects for success in the final fellowship exams, failed on the first day. The mental exhaustion and disappointment were palpable and severe: 'Broken wings' that had to 'learn to fly' again. This book is for all trainees in plastic surgery, junior and senior, but specifically for those who have had their wings broken. I was once one of them, and it took some years for me to 'take these sunken eyes and learn to see'.

No amount of study, mock (practice) exams or intensive training courses can really prepare the candidate for the reality of the final professional exams. This book, contributed to by invited experts and based on many years of clinical, educational and personal experience, may help to bridge the gap between preparation and the final test. We hope so.

The book is constructed as 16 chapters which cover the topics of psychology of examinations, digging yourself out of trouble, balancing acquired knowledge with bedside experience and the fundamental principles of plastic and reconstructive surgery.

The different segments of the exam are then dissected: Written papers, Long & Short clinical cases, Scenarios of Operative Surgery/Surgical Pathology and Gross Anatomy. Separate chapters then contrast the signs and symptoms of the successful versus the failing candidate. The final two chapters focus on general recommendations for exam preparation and summarise the body of the text with repetition and reinforcement.

Candidates should understand the attributes and calibre of the court of examiners that they will have to face. Examiners must have had at least 10 years of consultant plastic surgical experience and are invited to apply to the Court of Examiners of the Royal Australasian College of Surgeons. New examiners are approved by the current cohort of examiners and are selected for their wide spectrum of plastic surgical knowledge and clinical experience.

The mini-court of plastic surgery examiners is led by a senior examiner who has already had several years' experience as an examiner. The process of becoming an examiner involves a period of observation and mentoring by more experienced examiners. Examinations are generally conducted by a pair of examiners, and the pairings are rotated so that fairness and impartialness are the norm. The examiners are also scrutinised during the exam process, usually by senior examiners of the different surgical craft specialties and/or the Chair/Deputy Chair of the Court of Examiners. There is a process available to consider if a candidate feels discrimination or prejudice by an examiner. The examiners are also encouraged to declare any conflict of interest, and changes to the pairings will be organised by the senior examiner.

Despite what previous candidates may tell you, based on their personal experience, the exam process is very consistent, fair and transparent for all candidates from all surgical disciplines. The Court of Examiners constantly address issues of standardisation, educational validity and all other professional issues relating to the final exam process. Some candidates who are marginal but very close to a pass will have their case discussed anonymously in the presence of the Full Court of Examiners and a vote taken before the final mark is awarded.

Preparation, practice and perfecting your performance are the three key strategies for success in professional plastic surgery exams. When should you start? If you leave it to the last year of your advanced training (SET 5 *surgical education and training* in the RACS surgical training programme), you have given yourself a significant challenge. A common observation of supervisors of surgical training is that junior advanced trainees, after overcoming the battle and competition to win a place as a SET trainee, slip into comfortable 'cruise control'. It is our collective view that preparation for the final fellowship exam of the RACS should commence early in your plastic surgery training. Every new surgical technique, graft, flap and repair should be documented and important principles emphasised. Every outpatient clinic, ward round and operative session provides a rich tapestry of clinical data and personal experience that will help build your portfolio of knowledge, understanding and interpretation. These are the building blocks that will ultimately become the foundation of your surgical career, but also for the final exam.

In the modern world of work–lifestyle balance, it is mandatory to stay healthy and passionate during your training. To do this, some very simple fundamentals of self-care are emphasised:

Get to bed early (when not on duty), i.e. 10.30 pm at the latest.
Get 8 hours of quality sleep a night, if possible.
Get up early, i.e. 5.30–6.00 am.
Exercise every day, preferably in the mornings.
Drink plenty of water and not too much tea or coffee.
Eat well and choose lots of fruit and vegetables. Always have breakfast and lunch.
Learn to relax and develop an interest or hobby other than medicine.
Love your work and approach it with enthusiasm.
Respect your patients and your colleagues and strive to be a 'good doctor'.
Advocate for your patients, learn to be assertive but considerate.
Be strong, ask for help and always show compassion.
Your family always comes first, they need you.
Look after yourself.
Stay well, to practise well [1].

The Resilience Institute, founded by Dr Sven Hansen (a South African doctor), is an excellent resource. It has defined several practical solutions to enable body, hear and mind in your professional life, including how to avoid that sense of depression and helplessness caused by extreme pressure of work overload.

Dr Hansen lives by his own guidelines '*stay lean and fit, develop excellent sleep patterns and avoid sleep debt, eat lots of fruit, vegetables and fish, enjoy moderate amounts of red wine/blueberries/red grapes/beetroot, soy, beans, nuts, tomato and garlic additions to diet and finally learn and practice relaxation and mind rest*'.

Sleep is a key physiological function. Dr Hansen believes you should develop a relaxed and quiet hour or two before bedtime, i.e. prepare your mind and brain for quality sleep. Power naps for 10 min are also recommended when you are on the run and under the pump (a busy emergency on-call night). Try and wake up at a consistent time each day (early preferably) and spend at least 5 min stretching all your muscles. Dogs and cats do this routinely! 30 min of exercising is very beneficial in the mornings if you can build that into your schedule. Exercising at other times of the day is also very beneficial. In the evenings, if you are not on duty, make a point of disconnecting from work and switch to the home channel—engage with friends and family. Avoid the stimulation of television in that important hour before bedtime. Start to develop that quiet, mind preparation time.

Auckland, New Zealand	Michael F. Klaassen
Auckland, New Zealand	Earle Brown
June 2018	

References

1. Adapted from M. F. Klaassen in the self-published: *Some Wise Words from the 'Old Man'—advice from an old surgeon for his daughter beginning her internship 2010.*
2. Practical Resilience Book Series 2006. Sven.hansen@resiliencei.com

Acknowledgements

We acknowledge with appreciation the ideas, thoughts and contributions of Sophie Klaassen (Pre-FANZCA), Katherine Lanigan (FANZCA), Tom Marshall (BA), Michael Leung (FRACS), Katherine Scott and Henry Willis.

Sophie Klaassen is a senior anaesthetic trainee in Sydney, Katherine Lanigan is a consultant anaesthetist on the Central Coast, NSW, Tom Marshall is a clinical psychologist with the Canterbury DHB in Christchurch, Michael Leung is an Associate Professor of Plastic Surgery in Melbourne, Katerine Scott and Henry Willis are spouses and loved ones of anonymous examinees.

We would also like to acknowledge the collaboration and contributions of Dr. Mark Moore, AM, FRACS, fellow course tutor and Head of the Australian Craniofacial Unit in Adelaide.

Associate Professor Felix Behan, whose acronyms we have shared, is also acknowledged for his contributions.

We thank sincerely Dr. John Roy, FANZCA, a senior anaesthetist in the Bay of Plenty of New Zealand, who provided the exquisite macro photography, which graces the start of each chapter. He and the junior author have been a surgical/anaesthetic team for nearly 3 decades.

Finally, we thank all the patients and anonymous trainees, who courageously allowed us to share their images and innermost thoughts of exam experience. You have all now succeeded and for this we congratulate you.

Contents

About the Authors

Michael F. Klaassen, FRACS is a former examiner in plastic and reconstructive surgery with the Royal Australasian College of Surgeons (2000–2008) and a consultant plastic surgeon working in both New Zealand and Australia. For the past 8 years, he has convened the Auckland FRACS (Plast) Course with Earle Brown, FRCS, FRACS; Associate Professor Michael Leung, FRACS; and Dr Mark Moore, AM, FRACS. His special interest is in rehabilitating the failed candidate for whom he has a historical bond. There is very little published in this field, and this scarcity of resources was a motivating factor behind this book.

Earle Brown, FRCS, FRACS is a former Head of Plastic Surgery Unit/Clinical Director of Surgery at Middlemore Hospital, in Auckland, New Zealand. He mentored Michael Klaassen from the early 1980s and coached him to eventual success in the final fellowship exams for plastic and reconstructive surgery in 1989. Active in his retirement, Earle has continued as a tutor of computer science for his peer group and has been an enthusiastic member of the faculty for the Auckland FRACS (Plast) Course. He and Klaassen have also published books on the fundamentals of plastic surgery principles and local flap repair.

The Psychology of Exam Performance

Important Principles for Understanding What Determines a Successful Performance and How to Avoid Failure

1

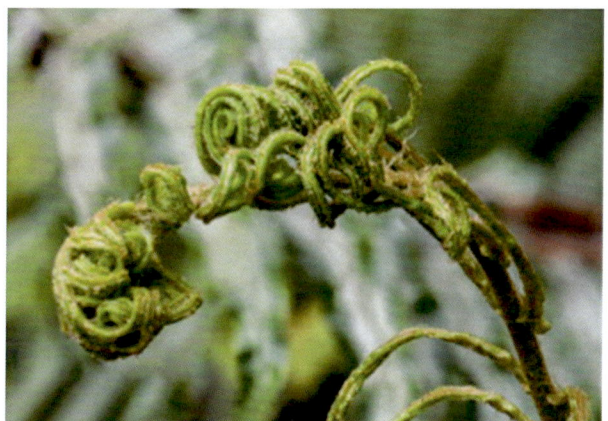

Fern

> *I have in my life concentrated more on self-expression than on self-denial.*
>
> (Winston Churchill, 1953)

> *Fearthought is futile worrying over what cannot be averted or will probably never happen.*
>
> (Winston Churchill, 1937).

Tom Marshall BA (Clinical Psychologist) contributed significantly to this first chapter.

© Springer Nature Singapore Pte Ltd. 2018
M. F. Klaassen and E. Brown, *An Examiner's Guide to Professional Plastic Surgery Exams*, https://doi.org/10.1007/978-981-13-0689-1_1

Plastic and Reconstructive Surgery is one of nine Surgical specialties, within the Royal Australasian College of Surgeons.

All of these Specialties are subject to a similar form of exit examination to qualify trainees for Specialist accreditation.

1.1   Surgical Specialties

Cardiothoracic Surgery
General Surgery
Neurosurgery
Orthopaedic Surgery
Otolaryngology/Head & Neck Surgery
Paediatric Surgery
Plastic & Reconstructive Surgery
Urology
Vascular Surgery

1.2   Preparing for the Right Exam

All surgical specialties have two professional exams. Part I consists of Basic Sciences and it is necessary to pass this before being accepted in to an accredited advanced surgical training program. Part I and part II exams are very different and preparation for them must be a balance of the required knowledge, surgical skill, experience, judgement and professionalism that is under analysis. This book is a guide to the final or exit professional plastic surgery exams, known in New Zealand and Australia as Part II or Final Fellowship Exams. Similar exams are set to meet the requirements at a consultant level of plastic surgery performance in other countries like UK, USA and Europe. It is mandatory that the candidate should be familiar with the content of the exam, the expectations of the examiners and the proposed exam schedules. These are all available via the internet and RACS (Royal Australasian College of Surgeons) website (www.surgeons.org). Instructions for exam candidates can also be found for a number of jurisdictions including the USA.

1.3   Performance: A Thought Experiment

A useful analogy for considering the big picture of final professional surgical exams is to imagine yourself, as an artist or actor performing on a floodlit stage in the darkened theatre. The examiners are the audience, visible and palpable, who are there to judge whether you are ready or not to progress with your surgical career. Over an 8-year period of continual observation and interaction with candidates, I as an examiner came to realise the important profile of the successful candidate and the stigmata of the failed candidate. This is covered in more detail in Chaps. 13 and 14 but overall the successful candidate is hardly ever outstanding. Rather they are universally competent, and exhibit good communication and sound clinical judgment. They are able to answer examiners' questions decisively, effectively and promptly. The problem candidate is nervous, a poor communicator, hesitant, lacking in confidence or over-confident with little insight. The abilities to organise your thoughts, verbalise your thinking and interact in a professional and safe manner are mandatory. Prioritisation of evidence in the history taking, good physical examination technique and assimilation of all the evidence in the immediate workup of a patient with a clinical problem are useful to practice and utilise.

1.4 There Are Some Do's and Don'ts in This Critical Performance

Never insult the examiners (e.g. One candidate seemed to object to answering questions from an examiner of the opposite gender).

Never argue with the examiners.

Never hurt a patient with rough exam technique (e.g. One candidate hurt a child whilst the child's lip was examined).

Never admit defeat midway through an oral exam (e.g. One candidate just gave up halfway through the anatomy viva, still stressed by what had been perceived rightly or wrongly, as a poor performance in the previous viva).

Never use an unorthodox method for physical examination (e.g. One memorable candidate examined a female patient's breasts for tumours, with the patient in the upright standing position!).

1.5 Important Similarities and Differences Between Exam Formats

This is particularly relevant to the different examination formats for written versus oral exams.

1.6 Limitations of Human Information Processing

There are some fundamental limitations of human information processing systems and these have implications for the candidate and the examiners. These will be considered from a productivity versus receptivity formula. There are some useful strategies to consider for managing these variables. Once understood these ideas can be used to improve the candidate's revision, preparation, practice and exam performance. See below in regard to the performance - arousal curve of candidate versus examiner conversations.

1.7   Maxim Number One

1.7.1   Engage Your Brain Before Your Mouth!

1.7.1.1 Checklist for Answers in Clinical and Oral (or Viva) Exams

This is a generic, hands-on checklist for preparing, organising and reviewing a verbally presented answer.

1. Understand the question. What is the essence of this question?
2. Scoping the answer—*how many points to be made?* Define the paramount principles in context.
3. Keep your answer to the subject.
4. Punchlines first—versus *conclusions and high mark value points.* Emphasise the key features, principles of management and keep it simple.
5. Should value be added to the literal answer?—*can you score extra marks by expanding on your answer beyond parameters of the question?*
6. Deciding how to finish the answer—*start and end well.*
7. Don't waffle.

1.7.1.2 How to Develop an Exam Preparation Methodology

This needs to be personalised, empirical and with appropriate feedback. Diagnosis and assessment of performance has been tested using simple, sophisticated audiovisual recording technology. Different methodologies have been applied including rehearsal scenarios, massed performance, exposure overlearning, state-dependent learning and mastery.

Consider organising yourself into study groups with peers who are similarly preparing for the exams. Practice on previous exam papers if they are available.

1.7.2   The Concept of Abstraction and Its Relevance to Exams

1.7.2.1 Building Repertoire of Roles

The importance and significance of shifting and transitioning between the roles of registrar/trainee and consultant plastic surgeon. How to think and talk like a consultant plastic surgeon?

1.7.2.2 The Performance/Arousal Curve

This has been defined from published studies in the psychological literature and demonstrates that the examiners are most alert at the beginning and the end of the examinees performance. Their concentration is the least in the middle segment of the viva interaction. If you start badly but improve during the performance, this may not be as advantageous as starting well and ending well, when the examiners will notice!

This has important implications for exam preparation and anxiety management.

1.7.2.3 The 'Hole in the Road'

The candidate should develop strategies for managing things which go amiss or turn into a 'catastrophe' during the exam. These situations include the realities of mental blockade, gaps in knowledge, misunderstanding an abiguous question, giving a wrong answer and then realising their error. The recovery strategy for this 'hole on the road' requires a generic and hands-on checklist to help minimise damage and gain control of the situation. Your recovery needs to reassure the examiners of your ability to get out of trouble.

1.7.2.4 Strategies for the Highly Anxious Candidate

Psychological counselling.
     Breathing/relaxation manoeuvres to control feelings of panic.
     Pharmacology and drug therapy for enhancing performance.

1.7.2.5 High Performance

The mental side of sporting performance has many parallels with the psychological aspects of professional surgical exam performance. No sportsperson has articulated this more clearly in recent times than the legendary New Zealand Rugby captain, Ricie McCaw [1]. His self-reflection which formed the basis of the 2016 movie/documentary *Chasing Great* by Justin Pemberton and Michelle Walsh explores a very personal insight into the captain's mind. This is an inspirational film which documents McCaw's struggle to come to terms with the challenges of handling pressure in elite sport. It analyses his approach to developing the capacity to control the mind in any stressful situation, particularly the dark places of intense battle and attrition in a World Cup Rugby final. The fear of defeat or failure can be viewed as either a Threat or a Challenge. By embracing the challenge head on, and developing mental toughness and conditioning, McCaw realised with the counselling of a forensic psychiatrist (Dr Ceri Evans) and other sports psychologists, he could learn how to overcome the challenge.

> The body will do what the mind says
> Richie McCaw (2016)

This was his most important role as captain of a winning international rugby team. The 2011 and 2015 back-to-back Rugby World Cup finals attest to this. Feeling on edge and nervous when challenged mentally and physically is a normal physiological/psychological reaction. The key strategies which McCaw realised he needed to have in his captain's toolbox, with which to confront the sporting challenges were:

Experience
Control
Composure
Discipline

Learning from your failures
Standing up for the challenge
Remaining focused

It is no different for the candidate faced with the challenge of final professional surgical exams, be they plastic surgery, cardiothoracic surgery, general surgery, neurosurgery, orthopaedic surgery, otolaryngology/head & neck surgery, paediatric surgery, urology or vascular surgery.

Reference

1. Pemberton J, Walshe M, Avery C. Chasing great (2016) – IMDb. www.imdb.com/title/tt5722234/

Caught in the Spotlight

2

Strategies for that Situation Where the Question is Very Challenging and You Feel Like a Rabbit Caught in the Glare of the Headlights

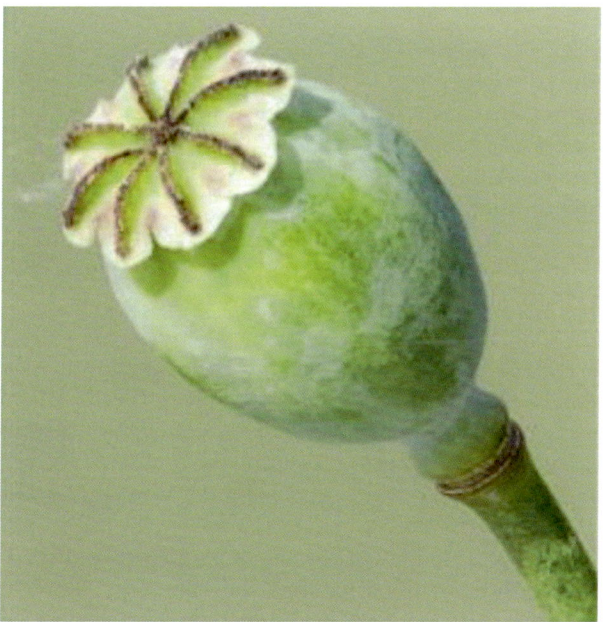

Opium Poppy Pod (Papaver somniferum)

> *In critical and baffling situations it is always best to recur to first principles and simple action.*
>
> (Winston Churchill, 1951)

This chapter considers that alarming situation where the candidate is faced with a written question, clinical scenario or actual long/short case, hitherto not encountered. They just do not have a clue? The critical strategy is to stay calm and alert, use all the senses of observation, description and logic to identify the broad category of

© Springer Nature Singapore Pte Ltd. 2018
M. F. Klaassen and E. Brown, *An Examiner's Guide to Professional Plastic Surgery Exams*, https://doi.org/10.1007/978-981-13-0689-1_2

what is the issue/problem/diagnosis? Jack Penn (1909–1996) and his son John Penn [1], both South African plastic surgeons wrote a paper in 1993 about generational differences and surgical principles, in which they concluded:

Basic principles last forever.
Simplicity is essential for well-planned and executed surgery.
Plastic surgery competence requires good taste and judgement.
There is nothing new under the sun.
The plastic surgeon is the composer and the virtuoso.

Dr. Jack Penn trained under the mentorship of Sir Harold Gillies, Archibald McIndoe, Rainsford Mowlem and Pomfret Kilner during the Second World War. He returned home to lead early plastic surgery in South Africa, where he established the Brenthurst Military Hospital for the plastic and reconstructive rehabilitation of the war wounded.

One of Sir Harold Gillies' first principles was *Observation is the key to surgical diagnosis.* His second principle, developed on the experience of thousands of war wounds, was *Diagnose before you treat.* These two principles are the starting points for when you are faced with a baffling situation. Keep it simple: what is the question really asking, what am I looking at here, what are the priorities? These are the questions that should automatically scroll through your consciousness. A candidate who is conversing during the viva voce is one who impresses the examiners.

The quiet candidate may in fact be a silent thinker, predisposed to this by their intrinsic character. The risk and reality, however, is that this comes across to the examiners as the ignorant candidate.

Remember that the examiner's concentration is peaking at the commencement and the final stages of the exam interaction. This was mentioned as the performance/arousal curve in the previous chapter. You should aim to start well and finish well. The concentration of the examiners will tend to wane during the middle of the session, they are human! A confident candidate will articulate their thoughts as they progress.

At the commencement of the Auckland FRACS Course for plastic surgery in 2015, I told the assembled group of candidates that they were the most inventive, creative, artistic and dedicated surgical trainees around. These are the young doctors we select for our advanced surgical programmes in Plastic & Reconstructive Surgery. Compliments are potentially encouraging but increasingly, the cohorts of trainees presenting for the coaching course require a wake-up call. I usually achieve this by telling them that when I was at their stage of career nearly 30 years ago, I failed the final fellowship exam twice … and I am still having nightmares about it. I wait for about five full seconds, see the blood drain from their faces and then add; 'just kidding!'

Encouragement and fear, nurturing and discipline, knowledge and experience, self-confidence and self-belief—these are the tools that we use to prepare the candidates for success in their professional exams.

Fig. 2.1 Mock question regarding breast reconstruction, in a 33-year-old woman after left mastectomy for invasive ductal carcinoma and staged reconstruction with tissue expansion and a latissimus dorsi flap

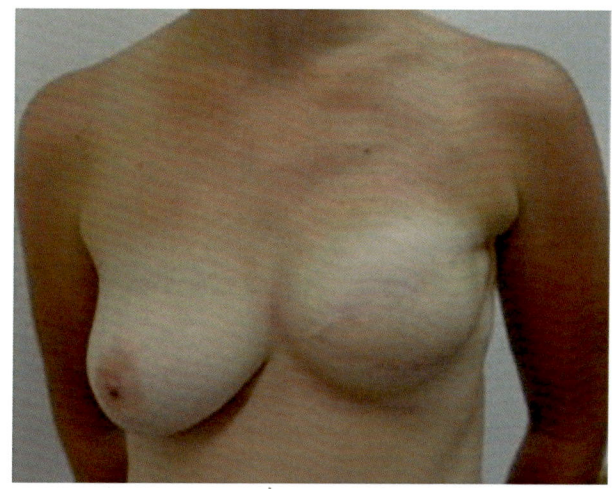

A number of mock (practice) and real exam scenarios experienced over the years come to mind.

The first is a mock question I set detailing the history of a 33-year-old woman, a marine biologist who presented with diffuse left breast ductal carcinoma in situ and a small focus of invasive carcinoma (Fig. 2.1). She had a full left mastectomy as advised by her breast surgeon and a year later was referred for consideration of breast reconstruction. Because of her wishes and lack of spare abdominal tissue, she underwent a staged left breast mound reconstruction with a latissimus dorsi myocutaneous flap over a tissue expander and once overexpansion had been achieved, a matched anatomical cohesive gel implant was inserted into the subpectoral-latissimus pocket. At this stage, she was 2 years post-breast cancer diagnosis and wanted to return to her career overseas. *She was very clear that she did not want a nipple–areolar reconstruction for the left side nor any modifications to the moderately ptotic contralateral normal breast.* Images of her pre-reconstruction and current reconstruction appearance were displayed. The question then asked the candidate: *Please discuss?*

This question based on the clinical scenario of one of my own patients has become a very reliable indicator of whether the candidate reads the question and answers it appropriately within context. Approximately, 90% of SET 5 registrars, preparing for the FRACS (Plast) final fellowship exam in the last 2 years, have failed it. They predictably launch into a long discussion of the imperfections of her left breast reconstruction, the asymmetry compared to the right moderately ptotic breast, the absence of the nipple–areola complex on the reconstructed left breast mound, the contour deficit in the lateral chest donor site and the scars. This is usually followed by an exhaustive list of possible further options including various free perforator flaps, fat grafting and mastopexy techniques.

The attentive, focused candidate, who has read the question carefully over and over, soon realises that this is not a question about breast reconstruction techniques. It is about listening to our patients, understanding their wishes, seeing the problem from their perspective and involving them in the team discussion, decisions and surgical planning. There is a raft of psychological research from Breast Cancer Care Teams that younger women with the challenge of breast cancer are more likely to worry about: breast cancer local recurrence, disease-free intervals and long-term survival than the subtle aesthetics of perfect breast symmetry, absence of the nipple–areola complex or absolutely matching inframammary fold levels. The patient in question was more concerned about returning to marine biology pursuits, getting married to her fiancé, having children, seeing them grow up and mature …. Being around to see them graduate, become adults, live fulfilling lives and more.

When the senior author was in practice, he used to tell breast reconstruction patients that the appearance of a reconstructed breast was never perfect. The minimum result was to have the shape and size equal to the opposite breast when wearing a bra. Most patients are accepting of these limitations and are more concerned with the oncological implications.

Mostly, the written questions will be more surgically focused, e.g. *Compare and contrast the surgical options for women with breast cancer presenting with normal* versus *high body mass indexes?* It is very helpful to the candidate and indeed the marking examiner, for a plan to be transcribed for the answer. This can be in bullet-point form, a series of headings, a diagram of interconnecting shapes (like an algorithm) or a concise summary as you would read in the abstract of a paper on a conference programme or published journal. The plan is the blueprint for your answer and shows the examiner that you have thought about it in a logical and constructive way (Fig. 2.2).

If you do not have a clue what the question is really about or what your answer should be, your plan could develop some intuitive lines of thought. What is the

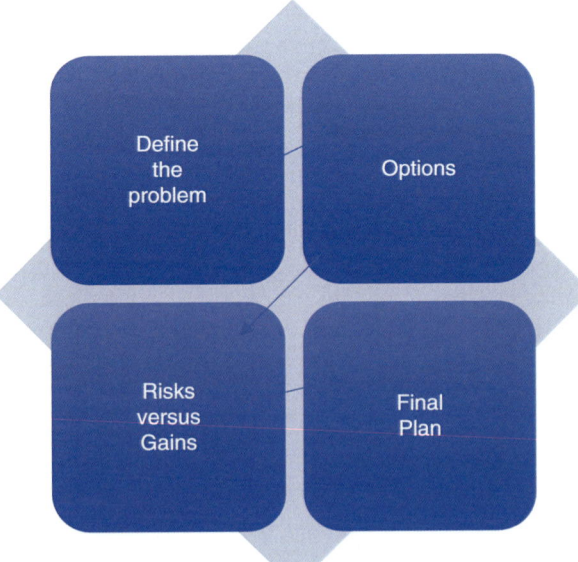

Fig. 2.2 Suggested plan for a model answer

differential diagnosis here? Are the management options critical from a timing perspective? Are there options that may be considered non-surgical? Can I manage this solo or do I require help from a multidisciplinary team of experts in their field? Do I need to speak with the referring general practitioner? What family support does the patient have that may influence her treatment choices? What does the patient fear, understand or expect? An important way to start is to connect with the patient or the problem and initiate a meaningful and constructive conversation where you, the doctor, show that you care for and respect them. Sir Archibald McIndoe taught another important principle which stated: *'Connectedness with your patient equals a confident trusting patient.'*

One of the first exams I ever examined in was when I was paired with the legendary Professor Wayne Morrison for the long cases at The Royal Children's Hospital in Melbourne. The first case was a toddler accompanied by his mother and he presented with a classic case of right-hand dominant radial club hand. I was nervous and did not expect such a rare first case. In the time that the paired examiners have to review the selected cases, before the candidates arrive, Wayne and I had the opportunity to assess the young patient. This was my moment of being caught like a hare in the oncoming headlights.

This is how I coped: general inspection and enquiry to rule out any other clinical issues, family history and genetic factors. Examination of both his upper limbs together, the left upper limb being a comparison for the right radial club hand. The position of his hand attached to his forearm in the radial deviated position was the obvious deformity but it was important to establish the movement and function of his elbow and movements of his hand to his mouth. The form and function of his thumb and digits was also a critical analysis. Radiology images were also available to help define his anatomy. The next appreciation after considering the history and physical findings was the timing of surgical correction, with paediatric orthopaedic collaboration, the risks associated with this, the future function of his right upper limb and hand dexterity and conversations with the mother about her understanding, concerns and fears. I realised pretty quickly that the principles of this deformity and its management were the key and not the fact that I had never encountered a case, even in my year of advanced orthopaedic training, nearly 20 years previously!

Fortunately, most of the presenting candidates that morning approached this long case with the same modus operandi and were successful.

Another example of a confronting difficult case which certainly tested many candidates attempting this mock written question in 2014 is illustrated (Fig. 2.3).

A 75-year-old retired secretary presents to your outpatient clinic with an ulcer of her left nasal vestibule. She is a chronic smoker with hypertension, atrial fibrillation and type 2 diabetes. The lesion has been present for at least 6 months and failed to respond to topical and oral antibiotics. **In 60 min discuss your plan of management and likely prognosis.**

Many candidates assumed that this was a basal cell carcinoma and offered inadequate surgical resection margins. The options for reconstruction in many cases were also on the conservative side with skin grafts and local flaps suggested.

Fig. 2.3 Nasal ulcer case, in a 75-year-old medical secretary with type 2 diabetes and a chronic smoker

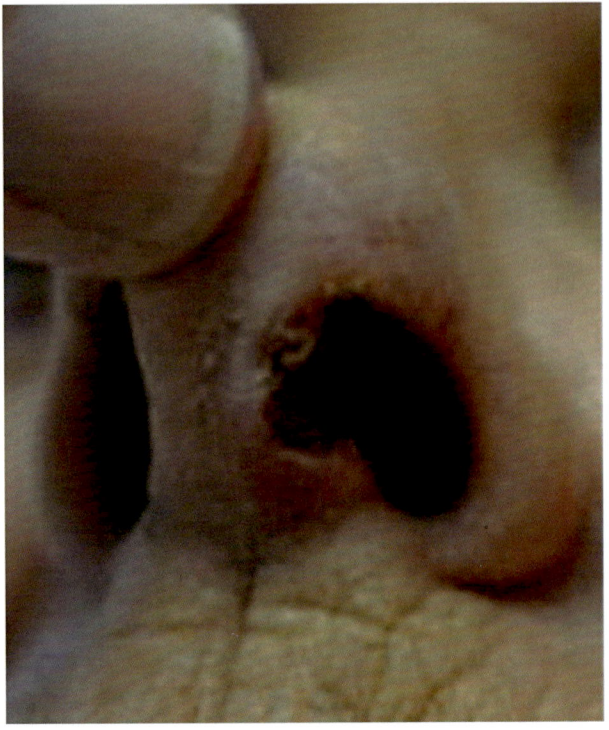

My initial observation of this clinical case would suggest an aggressive, penetrating squamous cell carcinoma of the nasal septum and columella in a heavy smoker with significant medical comorbidities. The lesion is at least 15 mm in diameter, ulcerated and examination should establish the clinical staging with examination of the contralateral nasal vestibule, nasal airway and hard palate for local tumour spread. Regional lymph node drainage basins should also be examined. The tumour should be biopsied for definitive pathological diagnosis and ideally a complete excision to establish clear margins. Delayed Reconstruction After Pathological Examination (DRAPE concept of Prof Felix Behan) and further imaging with CT/MRI are also mandatory. Ideally, these complex cases should be managed in a Multi-Disciplinary Team (MDT) setting such as a combined Head & Neck Cancer Clinic. After careful and professional workup, respecting the patient's wishes, definitive wide excision left a composite defect of the columella + caudal septum + nostril sill + left nasal vestibule. This was extended to include the nasal tip aesthetic subunit in order to achieve an aesthetic staged reconstruction (Aesthetica Concept—see Klaassen, Frame and Levick). Staged reconstruction ensued over several months with a forehead flap for cover, contralateral septal mucosal flap for lining and auricular cartilage grafts for structural support. Once reconstruction was completed, an opinion for adjuvant radiotherapy was requested.

The prognosis is related to the aggressiveness and local extent of the cancer but also on this patient's physiological status with respect to cardiac, respiratory and renal function. The issue of compliance is also relevant particularly with regard to the continuation of nicotine ingestion. Family support, socio-economic status, life expectancy and the patient's understanding of the important clinical and health issues must be considered in the doctor–patient conversations. These cases are complex for many reasons but can be summarised into what the patient really wants (usually survival and cure) and what is the appropriate management ethically, practically and realistically. Ultimately, her management was very successful and she remains healthy and well 4 years on.

Even if the candidate did not know the exact diagnosis for this case, a good start would be to verbalise and articulate their initial thoughts. State the obvious and what you see: *'This is a tumour of the nasal septum extending into the nasal tip'*. Avoid jumping into a diagnosis straight off if you are uncertain. Play for some time whilst your brain is processing all the evidence by leading the examiners in your conversation. You could be describing the detailed features and morphology of the tumour, pigmentation or lack of, show them your competent understanding of the anatomy of the particular region—the layers of structures (skin, cartilage and mucosal lining) and the associated regional anatomy (nasal airway, upper lip, paranasal sinuses, regional lymph node basins and aesthetic nasal subunits).

Even after years of clinical practice, the experienced plastic surgeon will encounter clinical problems never before seen. I work with a number of other surgical colleagues including urologists and gynaecologists. Two quite different clinical cases referred to me by them recently included a young man with Squamous Cell Carcinoma of the glans penis, associated with psoriasis, and a middle-aged woman with a lateral left flank bulge following left partial nephrectomy and complicated by irreversible damage to the left subcostal nerve. If I had been recruiting long clinical cases for a forthcoming exam, then these two challenging examples would have been ideal. Let us now consider them individually.

2.1 Long Case 01: Carcinoma of the Glans Penis

Long history of chronic psoriasis, immunosuppression and erythematous plaque-like lesions (SCC in situ*) on glans penis of a young man. Recent biopsy confirmed invasive well-differentiated SCC involving 2 cm area on the dorsum of the glans. Lesion extends close to but not into the external urethral meatus. No palpable inguinal lymphadenopathy.*

This is an unusual presentation in my experience but the principles of plastic surgery define the best course of action. Collaboration with the referring urologist is ideal. The diagnosis is clear cut with available biopsy results and if the nodes are clear, (based on lymphoscintigraphy) then the TNM classification is T2, N0, M0 and the lesion is stage 1. Treatment in this situation involves a wide local excision, preservation of the urethra, aesthetic reconstruction with a full thickness skin graft and elective sentinel node biopsy. Partial resection of the glans is obviously a potentially disfiguring and very threatening reality for the patient, so counselling about the indications to achieve complete local excision and immediate aesthetic reconstruction is important. There will be tissue missing so replacement is an important reconstructive consideration. A thick split skin graft or thin full thickness skin graft will provide the most durable cover, rather than a preputial flap (if he is uncircumcised). There will be the need to bypass the urine stream with an indwelling catheter, whilst vascularisation of the skin graft is occurring over the first 5–7 days. Immobilisation of the graft with a tie-over dressing and medications to suppress nocturnal penile erections should also be considered. The question of more radical surgery such as distal penectomy could be mentioned but the favourable histology reported probably favours less radical resection (partial dorsal glansectomy) and functional preservation. In the medium term, the consideration of distal meatal stenosis could be predicted and serial dilatations required to prevent urinary flow obstruction.

2.1.1 Guiding Principles Case 01

Diagnosis
Staging
Complete Local Excision + Aesthetic Reconstruction (CLEAR)
If CLEAR not possible, then Delayed Reconstruction After Pathological Examination
   (DRAPE)
Consideration of complications—perioperative, early and late

2.2   Long Case 02: Lateral Abdominal Hernia

Middle-aged woman referred by her urologist with a lateral abdominal bulge for 5 years following partial left nephrectomy for an oncocytoma. She is self-conscious of it despite her otherwise high body mass index and wants to have her abdominal contour restored to 'normal'. She also experiences back pain which she associates with the lateral abdominal bulge.

An upper lateral abdominal hernia secondary to partial nephrectomy and subcostal nerve injury is rare. The commonest complications from this type of surgery could be infection, haemorrhage, transient ischaemia associated with this technique and renal insufficiency. Damage to the left subcostal nerve is either overt during the sharp dissection or more likely from traction by the wound retractors. Examination of the patient in the reclined and upright postures reveals <u>at least</u> a 10 × 10 cm muscular weakness in her left abdominal wall associated with a positive cough reflex. Palpation should also reveal any pulsatile mass. It would be appropriate to consider the relevant anatomy, aware of anatomical anomalies and associated structures. The subcostal nerve is derived from the anterior ramus of the 12th thoracic nerve, which travels through the abdominal musculature to innervate external oblique and rectus abdominis. Its sensory innervation is to the skin lateral to the ASIS (anterior superior iliac spine) of the pelvic brim. These are easily tested by examination. Associated neighbouring nerve structures could be mentioned to demonstrate your anatomical knowledge viz. the iliohypogastric (T12-L1), ilioinguinal (L1) and genitofemoral (L1-L2) trunk nerves. The status of her renal tumour is of some importance. What is the risk of recurrence and is there potential for other oncocytomas? This is a benign tumour of epithelial cells occurring in the kidney and the conservative approach of partial nephrectomy to spare nephrons and avoid chronic renal insufficiency is the treatment of choice. Conversations and collaboration with the patient's urologist would be mandatory in regard to any future surgery such as hernia repair. Oncocytomas can occur in any organ and may have a premalignant potential. The management of her flank hernia depends on a preanaesthetic workup, radiological imaging and dietary advice to reduce her high BMI to a level that is compatible with safe elective surgery.

Repair of the abdominal hernia needs to consider the following options:

1. Direct previous incision approach versus midline approach.
2. Extraperitoneal dissection and delineation of the hernia boundaries.
3. Repair with alloplastic (mesh) or autogenous (musculofascial) methods.
4. Postoperative management early and medium-term to protect the repair and maximise respiratory function (risk of raised intra-abdominal pressure).
5. Combined surgical approach of urological & plastic surgeons.

I personally favour the use of autogenous tissues for repair if possible and avoidance of mesh or similar foreign bodies. The availability of external oblique fascia, fascia lata grafts from her thighs and pedicled muscular flaps such as a reverse latissimus dorsi flap could all be considered in the surgical plan.

2.2.1   Guiding Principles Case 02

Defining the status of her tumour, risk of recurrence and associated tumours.
Imaging of the left lateral retroperitoneal hernia with MRI or CT.
Planning a repair via a midline approach, extraperitoneal dissection.
Deciding which autogenous musculofascial tissues are available locally for strong repair of the hernia with or without mesh.
Careful anaesthetic workup for perioperative care and post-operative recovery.

2.3   Summary: Caught in the Spotlight

1. Read, listen and understand the questions.
2. Always define the diagnosis—*diagnose before your treat*.
3. Consider the diagnostic ladder: *Congenital, Traumatic, Neoplastic, Metabolic, Inflammatory (CTNMI)*.
4. Have a plan and some options—*make a plan and a pattern*.

5. Fall-back position is first principles and simplicity.
6. Define the relevant anatomy.
7. Always have a plan B—*have a lifeboat.*
8. Consider the trilogy—*what could I do, what do I want to do and what should I do?*
9. If there is a less complex option, choose it.
10. Seek help—*ask colleagues for second opinions.*
11. Do not let routine method become your master—*Gillies.*
12. Do not be afraid to be bold, take responsibility for the surgical challenge and do what is in the best interests of the patient and their family.
13. Embrace the challenge of this 'dark place', stay calm, composed and focused.

Reference

1. Penn JG, Penn J. Reflections on two generations in plastic surgery. Plast Reconstr Surg. 1993;91(4):718–9.

Knowledge Is Power, Experience Is Key

3

How to Balance the Wealth of Knowledge Gained from Reading with the Wisdom of Surgical Experience

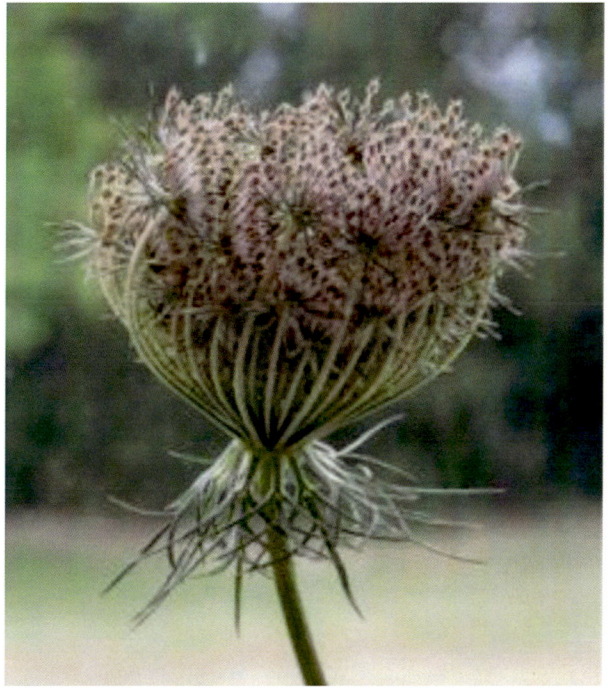

Daucus

The only source of knowledge is experience.

(Albert Einstein)

© Springer Nature Singapore Pte Ltd. 2018
M. F. Klaassen and E. Brown, *An Examiner's Guide to Professional Plastic Surgery Exams*, https://doi.org/10.1007/978-981-13-0689-1_3

Senior plastic surgery trainees presenting for the final fellowship examination have probably more knowledge about the scope and theory of plastic and reconstructive surgery than at any other stage of their surgical careers. They may be limited in their knowledge of aesthetic surgery and some other subspecialties of the discipline but what they really lack is experience, i.e., the experience of thinking, planning and operating at a consultant level of competence. This is inevitable given that the previous 4–5 years have largely been a professional working life as a junior team member, with a supervising consultant or mentor above them. The final professional exams are predominantly about demonstrating through a series of confrontational interactions with experienced surgeon examiners that they are ready to make the step up to be a junior consultant. Dr. Sean Hamilton FRACS a former senior examiner for the Court of Examiners (RACS) used to emphasise that from his perspective 'If the situation presented it, could this candidate he was examining be capable of taking over his practice for the next six weeks if he was temporarily out of action through illness, absence or other unexpected circumstance'? In other words, could the candidate step into his shoes?

This chapter considers the broad range of the plastic surgery curriculum against the spectrum of clinical knowledge, decision-making, judgement and appropriate surgical management. It can be categorised into what is possible, what could I do and more importantly what should I do? The categories of knowledge fall into predictable and examinable topics including: adult and paediatric diagnoses, trauma, cancer and reconstructive and aesthetic surgery. The following categories will be considered in more detail:

Facial and neck rejuvenation (Aesthetic Surgery Principles)
Periorbital rejuvenation
Craniofacial surgery (Craniofacial Surgery Principles including those for cleft lip and palate + associated anomalies, orthognathic surgery)
Microsurgery (Reconstructive Principles for free tissue transfer, replantation, brachial plexus surgery)
Breast surgery (Principles of breast reduction, mastopexy, augmentation and reconstruction of the breast)
Ear reconstruction (including non-surgical methods of neonatal ear molding)
Vascular anomalies
Tissue expansion
Fat grafting
Minimally invasive aesthetic procedures
LASER and chemical peels
Endoscopic and minimally invasive surgery
Hand and upper limb surgery
Lower limb and foot surgery

3.1   Aesthetic Surgery of the Face

Every patient wanting a facelift has a hidden agenda (Patrick Jerome Beehan FRACS)

Rejuvenation of the face includes the brow, eyelids, midface, lower face and neck. A variety of methods can be applied from minimalist conservative to advanced extended deep plane dissection and combining this with fat grafting (lipomorphoplasty), bone augmentation with hydroxyapatite, endoscopic instrumentation and topical therapies to the skin texture and tone (chemical, LASER and intense pulsed light). A comprehensive understanding of the pathophysiology of facial ageing is mandatory and this has been well documented over the last 100 years. Cultural and ethnic differences should also be appreciated (Caucasian, Asian, Polynesian, African, Middle-Eastern and mixed racial groups). Historically, the evolution of facelifting began in the nineteenth century with skin only, minimalist lifts then over the twentieth century the discovery of the deep facial planes, SMAS layer and retaining fascial ligaments lead to ever-increasing deep plane dissections and various facelift vectors. In the last 20 years, there has been a return to the minimalist techniques contrasted with more refinement of the extended techniques. Associated with this has been a renewed interest in three-dimensional form and contours, natural facial spaces that allow safe access to the key retaining ligaments and the combined use of neurotoxins and dermal fillers to augment the ageing face. Beyond the surgical techniques, there exist the fundamental issues of aesthetic facial surgery including motivations, agendas, expectations, personalities and psychological issues which may appear to be a minefield to the novice. In reality, experience with patients hones the surgeon's intuitive understanding of what the real agenda is. Conversations, documentation, 'cooling off' periods and detailed consideration of the surgical risks are essential. *How long does a facelift last?* This is a critical question that Barry Jones FRCS et al. attempted to answer in a key paper [1].

Patients need to understand that ageing is progressive, despite rejuvenative surgery of any method and some patients will require maintenance corrections. The loose neck is one significant problem that can return.

Restoring a youthful neck in harmony with a rejuvenated face has specific challenges. The neck is by nature a mobile structure, carrying the head and face and anatomically inseparable, in more ways than one! Many patients notice the ageing of their neck as a primary stigma and want this corrected. It is difficult to change one without the other. The platysma muscle is the key anatomical feature closely related to its cephalad extension of the SMAS layer. Modifications of the fat layer in the neck also become surgical options with any combination of resection, liposuction or lipofilling. The neck skin remodelling and redraping should be approached with the goal of producing an attractive neck. This should keep in mind the lower neck with the distinctive suprasternal notch—often ignored as noticed by Hodgkinson [2].

The youthful neck ideally also defines the whole of the sternomastoid muscle deep to platysma from mastoid process to the suprasternal notch. The platysma–SMAS complex and its importance to facial aesthetics has been recognised since the earliest writings of perhaps the world's greatest anatomist Andre Vesalius, in his sixteenth century treatise De humani corporis fabrica [3].

Vesalius referred to it as the fleshy membrane extending from the clavicles to the cranium. Hodgkinson has noted the fascial attachments of platysma including the well-defined auriculoparotid ligament (prelobar fascia), the contested fascial attachments to the anterior border of the mandible and to the hyoid bone. The primary attachments of platysma are to the skin of the neck but there exists a loose areolar plane deep to platysma, which can be entered surgically and allows for considerable sliding of the platysma vertically without distortion of the neck strap muscle or sternomastoid muscle. These anatomical details allow for correction of the sagging platysma and platysmal bands. Hodgkinson's modification of Fogli's fixation of platysma to Lore's fascia achieves a lower and more anterior fixation of platysma muscle which can address primarily or secondarily the ageing neck features. Technical details aside, the student of plastic surgery is wise to appreciate the subtle anatomical details described above. The improved youthfulness of Hodgkinson's published series speak for themselves. This surgical thinking is a convenient addition to the armamentarium of the occasional facelift surgeon, in particular, the relatively inexperienced examination candidate.

3.2   Periorbital Rejuvenation

Upper blepharoplasty has evolved in recent times to a phase of more conservative management avoiding excessive extraorbital fat resection (with the risk of bleeding and retrobulbar haematoma) and correction of associated ptosis with techniques to anchor the upper tarsal plate to the levator aponeurosis and margin of the orbicularis oculi muscle. The relatively simple anchor blepharoplasty as described by Flowers et al. from Hawaii produces very natural rejuvenated results and can be achieved with local anaesthetic only. In assessing the patient with excess upper eyelid skin and dermatochalasia, consideration should always be given to the contribution of brow ptosis and the need to combine upper blepharoplasty with browlift or browpexy.

The lower eyelid ageing features with bagginess and weakening of the septum orbitale are more challenging and the lower eyelid as an anatomical structure less forgiving when overcorrected. Techniques to correct these problems include careful and balanced resection of lower eyelid skin ('Pinch' blepharoplasty), tightening of the orbital fascial septum and even the release of the septum and the infraorbital fat pads to reset the infraorbital contours as described by Hamra et al. Any discussion of lower eyelid blepharoplasty should consider the complication of lower eyelid retraction and ectropion. Methods to correct this are useful and require experience and careful timing. The timeless principles of Gillies come to mind, especially his *'Don't do today what can be honourably put off until tomorrow.'* Patience, time and masterly inactivity with massage, stretching of immature scars and the use of injectable Triamcinolone can buy valuable time. The lower eyelid–cheek junction is a special challenge where midface approaches and judicious lifting and periosteal fixation can get the surgeon 'out of jail'.

3.3 Craniofacial Surgery Principles

These have been defined very clearly by Mark Moore AM, FRACS, Head of the Australian Craniofacial Unit, Adelaide and should be considered as the continuum from childhood to adulthood. Craniomaxillofacial surgery should be encompassed in an appreciation of craniofacial surgery principles including the subspecialty of orthognathic surgery addressing facial form, the dental occlusion and significantly the airway. This super-specialised branch of plastic surgery includes the principles for the team-lead, protocol-based strategies for cleft lip and palate, hemifacial microsomia, ear reconstruction and rare conditions such as craniofacial neurofibromatosis and fibrous dysplasia. Orthognathic surgery remains one of the most powerful tools to change the appearance of the human face as well as improvement in the airways of selected cases.

3.4 Reconstructive Microsurgery

Like craniofacial surgery, reconstructive microsurgery has significant global networks pioneered by centres of excellence like the Bernard O'Brien Microsurgery Institute at Melbourne's St Vincent's Hospital and Chang Gung Memorial Hospital in Taiwan. The operating microscope and free tissue transfer techniques have heralded the growth in replantation surgery (hand, limb and face), brachial plexus surgery, toe-to-hand transfer, long bone reconstruction and mandibular reconstructions. Historically, a missionary doctor Dr. Sam Nordhoff pioneered this advance back in the late 1950s, selecting young and talented surgeons such as Fu-Chan Wei (microsurgery) and Yu-Ray Chen (craniofacial surgery) and sending them abroad for advanced training. The thousands of cases successfully performed by these modern world leaders of plastic surgery defy belief and have set the standard for the rest of the world. The surgical techniques have been honed in parallel with careful research to define the use of the vascularised fibular flap (VFF) for bone transfer, the modern free perforator flap (intramuscular dissection of pedicles), jejunal transfer for oesophagus and voice reconstruction, brachial plexus and functioning muscle transfer for limb and facial palsy reconstruction, vascularised joint transfer and limb and face transplantation. Clinical service, education and training and research have always been the three key drivers.

3.5 Breast Surgery Principles

A holistic approach to the patient with breast deformity, cancer and congenital anomalies should be equally considered for the reconstructive and aesthetic needs of the modern breast patient. These range from the twentieth century description of latissimus dorsi as a workhorse by Tansini and Olivari, the TRAM flap of Hartrampf to the microsurgery application of the free abdominoplasty flap by Hamilton and Fogdestam. The goals should include the complete local excision of the breast cancer and aesthetic reconstruction (CLEAR) either immediately, delayed or staged according to the individual needs of the breast patient. Autogenous tissue, prosthetic implants, tissue expansion and fat grafting have all evolved as the many and varied options available to the breast oncoplastic surgeon. Team-based approaches with the collaboration of medical and radiation oncologists supported by psychologists and breast care nurses provide a skilled and multidisciplinary approach to the modern management of breast cancer.

The evolving techniques from the nineteenth to the twenty-first centuries, from simply partial mastectomies to the goal of aesthetic refinement, preservation of form and function, have seen increasingly significant contributions from the female members of the plastic surgery community, led by Lejour, Hall-Finlay and Graf. An evolving morality and awareness of the importance of breast morphology from the female body image perspective may still to this day mean that aesthetic and reconstructive breast surgery is misunderstood.

Dr. Madeleine Lejour (1983) once commented that reduction of the hypertrophic breast with or without mastopexy is perhaps the most difficult form of breast surgery.

'C'est. peut-etre la plus difficile des formes de chirurgie mammaire ...'
                                                                                Dr. Madeleine Lejour

3.6   Ear Reconstruction

This very human of facial appendages can be considered from anotia, to microtia to the multiple deformations encountered from birth to childhood. The Japanese have led the way in the methods of neonatal ear molding for common and rare ear deformations (including ear prominence, lop ear and various helical deformities). Ear molding for a number of deformations was popularised by Gault and Tan in London in the 1990s. The earlier molding commences the shorter the time required to achieve correction of the deformation. Babies seen early in the first week or two perhaps need only 2–3 weeks of molding. Older children from 3–6 months require up to 12 or more weeks of molding. Commercially available EarBuddies can be used or tailor-made splints from lead-free soldering wire wrapped in Fixomull tape and fitted to the ear with Steristrips, Micropore or more Fixomull. The technique of neonatal ear molding is simple, effective and in my hands over the past 7 years has produced more natural-looking ears than any method of surgical otoplasty.

The standard methods of staged ear reconstruction pioneered by Dr. Burt Brent (USA) using constructions of autologous rib cartilage, and the emergence of new prosthetic materials like Medpor (? PGA) are now being challenged by the improvements in tissue engineering technology. The Chinese group led by Dr. Yilin Cao have developed chondrocyte tissue engineering of a PGA/PLA template designed with a 3D printer and using bone marrow stem cells and microtia remnant chondrocytes to create a soft auricular shell and framework, which can be covered with temporal fascia and expanded postauricular skin. The results require a special skill set, experience and persistence but are setting new standards in aesthetic ear reconstruction. For units not having this expertise, the alternative method of osseointegrated prosthetic implants based on the Swedish Brånemark technology offers alternative management options.

3.7   Vascular Anomalies

Haemangiomas and vascular malformations are common topics in plastic surgery exams. The understanding and cell biology of these relatively common paediatric conditions has grown rapidly in recent years with the discovery of placenta-origin stem cells and the renin–angiotensin pathways which control their proliferation. Tan et al. at the Gillies McIndoe Research Institute in Wellington, New Zealand have led the revolution in this progress. Fifty percent of haemangiomas in a child will involute by the age of five and 70% by the age of 7 years. For functionally disabling haemangiomata, for example intraorbital lesions and lesions obstructing the aerodigestive tract, beta blockers and calcium channel blocking drugs from the cardiology field, given in specific doses with close clinical monitoring, produce excellent resolution, without surgery. For low flow vascular malformations, the pulsed dye LASER has a role, particularly for the disfiguring facial port wine stain. For the more challenging high flow vascular malformations, intravascular treatment with sclerosants such as ethanol and other embolic agents applied by interventional radiologists achieve effective embolisation which can be followed with surgical resection. These potentially life-threatening lesions require management by Multi-Disciplinary Teams in centres of excellence. Sclerotherapy and ligation suture techniques have also been used and Tanner et al. in England have led this approach. Arteriovenous malformations can be very challenging to manage but very good results have now been achieved combining embolisation and complete surgical resection. The complications are significant but facial function especially that of the seventh cranial can be preserved. Sometimes, uncontrollable haemorrhage necessitates these lesions being managed in the emergency scenario.

3.8   Tissue Expansion

The use of carefully selected and anatomically placed expandable implants using saline, air or self-expanding devices which absorb body fluids offers a method for reconstruction in the restoration of scalp, facial, breast, trunk and limb defects. Nowhere has this been more effective clinically, than in the management of giant naevi of the scalp, face and trunk. The Chinese have been using this effectively since 1984 and pioneers like Jiang Li are now using multiple new tissue expanders with external ports, capable of volumes from 400 to 1000 cc. The potential problems with patient compliance are something the Chinese have overcome and their results with long-term follow-up, particularly in the field of late burn scar reconstruction, are truly amazing.

3.9   Fat Grafting

Sydney Coleman from New York reinvented the technique of Lipostructure™, lipo-morphoplasty and fat grafting in the mid-1990s, as a response to the challenge of complications resulting from the use of retroviral drugs in the war against HIV and Aids. Recent research has raised the question about the potential problem of ligno-caine causing the lysis of fat cell grafts and practitioners like Lee Pu from California advise the use of low concentration lignocaine (e.g. 0.05%). This may be an in vitro phenomenon and may not have the same clinical risk. Refinement of fat grafts har-vested by sedimentation, centrifuging or rinsing in saline all have their promoters. Delicate, atraumatic handling of the harvested fat grafts would seem to be the pre-vailing principle. The fat grafts harvested from the lower abdomen and inner thighs have more stem cells than other sites and should be the primary donor sites for suc-cessful outcomes. Overcorrection with refined fat grafts from these ideal donor sites does not seem to be necessary, although Coleman himself still practices a degree of overcorrection to counter the risk of absorption of some grafts. Blunt cannulae for the placement of fat grafts in small increments/aliquots layer by layer to achieve volume restoration are safer than sharp needles. For aesthetic facial rejuvenation with fat grafts, the volume of fat injected can vary from case to case, but as a guide volumes of 12–30 cc of fat are usual. I have personally used 80 cc for a middle-aged woman with severe fat atrophy. Small volume fat grafting is the norm for facial rejuvenation (<100 cc), whereas large volume fat grafting (100–200 cc) is best for the breast and body. Parry–Romberg's disease (hemifacial atrophy) is a reconstruc-tive indication for fat grafting in selected cases, as are post-radiation damage and post-traumatic contour defects. A new and alarming potential complication reported in the USA for temporal and periorbital fat grafting is blindness and two cases were reviewed by Dr. Gregory Evans in 2016. There have also been deaths reported from large volume fat grafting of the buttocks and the rare cases of intravascular injection of fat grafts in the face leading to ischaemic necrosis.

3.10   Minimally Invasive Aesthetic Procedures

Botox (Botulinum Toxin A) is a neuromodulating therapy for reducing wrinkle lines by selective blockade of the skeletal muscle motor endplates. This product also blocks the secretory skin glands and enhances skin volume by reducing microfluid loss.

Fillers (non-fat)

Non-fat injectables such as Hyaluronic Acid (HA) have also been associated with irreversible blindness in China. This may be related to non-medical use of injectables by untrained individuals capitalising on recent boom in Chinese cos-metic procedures. In this country, the use of non-fat Dermal fillers and HA, greatly exceeds that of fat grafting. Arterial embolisation is a severe complication particu-larly into the branches of the ophthalmic artery where partial, temporary or perma-nent blindness can be the outcome. There are ten potential branches of the ophthalmic artery with connections to the facial artery so the periorbital and paranasal regions are the most dangerous. Arterial injection is a potential risk within 30 min of the injection presenting clinically as severe pain and immediate blindness. Immediate ophthalmological evaluation is mandatory and if there is no blood flow within 90 min then permanent blindness will result. Prevention is the key and special training and experience are the prerequisites for safe practice and reducing complications.

3.11   LASER and Chemical Peels

LASER technology is constantly evolving and applications are considered in skin resurfacing for rejuvenation and tightening of the dermal layer. It can also be used as a cutting tool for superficial skin cancers and actinic damage. Some basic physics should be appreciated for the principles of LASER technology from the perspective of different wavelengths and the range of lesions that are treatable from photodamage, superficial rhytids, port wine stains, tattoos (acquired and traumatic) and the use of combined therapies (facelift surgery + LASER resurfacing). LASER technology has been adapted for high energy-based liposuction and also for the application of TORS (Trans-Oral Robotic Surgery).

The historic development of chemical peels is interesting and relevant. The early non-medical peelers of Las Vegas in the 1930s influenced the acceptance of this method for facial rejuvenation with the combined use of Phenol + Croton oil as pioneered by Baker and Gordon. More recently, Dr. Richard Bensimon [4] of Oregon has popularised the use of varying strength Croton oil peels, which require special training in both the preparation and the application clinically. The long-term results for facial rejuvenation in all racial skin types are quite impressive but the major challenge is the considerable downtime for the patient with the acute desquamation and the persisting erythema, which can last for several weeks and months.

3.12   Endoscopic and Minimally Invasive Surgery

The surgical endoscope has defined its place in plastic surgery predominantly in the field of brow rejuvenation. Some recent champions of endoscopic facial surgery such as Dr. Jung Wu of Taiwan are now combining this with minimally invasive scissor dissection for the neck. Through postauricular and low occipital incisions, the endoscopic instruments can be used to precisely dissect the supra-SMAS/platysma layers. The main advantages seem to be visual and magnification. Modified instruments with flatter, more obtuse angles enable also the more common brow and periorbital subperiosteal endoscopic dissection, ligament release and then fixation of the repositioned soft tissues with bone anchors or miniscrews. The Endotine device is a multiple point fixation device that is implanted into the calvarium for browlift and midface lifts. The main contraindication for my cohort of patients is the need for a general anaesthetic and the costs of endoscopic equipment and fixation devices. Personally, I do not favour the extensive dissections required based on the principle that the more dissection and tissue damage equals the more long-term tissue atrophy and exaggerated facial ageing. Minimally invasive surgeries utilising various endoscopes and laparoscopes have been applied for access to facial fractures and for the endoscopic dissection of flaps such as latissimus dorsi. Robotic surgery has been applied in the Head and Neck Cancer field for TORS (Trans-Oral Robotic Surgery) in the resection of parapharyngeal and other head and neck malignancies. This new technology offers more precision, less invasive surgery and functional preservation.

3.13   Hand and Upper Limb Surgery

A range of hand and upper limb clinical conditions cover the spectrum from congenital anomalies and acquired conditions such as inflammation, cancer and trauma. From an exam perspective, paediatric conditions such as syndactyly, thumb hypoplasia and obstetric palsies are likely to be sourced for clinical vivas. Adult hand conditions could include: burn contractures, major peripheral nerve palsies including the brachial plexus, radial, ulnar and median nerve palsies, Dupuytren's disease and various hand tumours (ganglia, neuromas and bone cysts). It is important to have a thorough knowledge of applied hand and upper limb anatomy, specific examination skills that test particular functions such as power and precision grip, fine motor skills and joint dysfunction. Phalen's test for carpal tunnel compression, Bouvier's test for intrinsic minus demonstration and Finkelstein's test for De Quervain's tenosynovitis are just some of these. The applied anatomy knowledge is also important for the use of various reconstructive flaps for the hand and upper limb. The keystone perforator island local flap (Behan) and the Radial Forearm loco-regional/distant fasciocutaneous or osteofasciocutaneous flaps would be my workhorse flaps for upper limb. Intimate knowledge of their applied anatomy and variations of flap design are critical for the clinical oral exams including the anatomy exam.

A comprehensive appreciation of hand and upper limb surgery includes an understanding of the role of the hand physiotherapist, occupational therapist, pain management team and other experts contributing to the rehabilitation team.

3.14   Lower Limb and Foot Surgery

Over the many years that I have been involved in professional plastic surgery exams, the clinical topic of chronic osteomyelitis has always been a popular theme. The aetiologies, pathophysiology and principles of surgical management of chronic bone infection, should be essential knowledge to the young plastic surgeon. Other challenging conditions such as the various spinal injuries and neurological conditions like multiple sclerosis, Guillaine–Barre syndrome and diabetic peripheral neuropathies, with their sequelae including decubitus ulcers, and chronic wound healing difficulties are also considered. The key flaps for me starting from the toes and progressing to the proximal thigh are: various great toe transfers for thumb reconstruction, the extensor digitorum brevis local muscle flap, the medial plantar fasciocutaneous flap, the reverse sural artery fasciocutaneous flap, the medial and lateral gastrocnemius muscle flaps, the multiple keystone perforator island local flaps either singly, doubly or with the variants of Yin Yan, Omega or bespoke. The anterior thigh fasciocutaneous flap offers large surface cover. The traditional groin flap, tensor fascia lata, hamstring and buttock musculocutaneous flaps still have their important and specific uses too (see Chap. 9).

Another favourite and recurring exam topic in this anatomical region is lymphoedema. One of the leading experts in the field of lymphoedema and its management is Dr. Hung-Chi Chen of Taiwan. Correct diagnosis is important because 90% of lymphoedema cases can be treated with conservative measures. When fibrosis is established then surgery is indicated and these are the remaining 10% of cases. The surgical options include modifications of the traditional Charles Procedure (excisional, 1912) and more modern drainage versus excisional procedures. Lymph node transfer (gastroepiploic lymph node flap) is achieved by microsurgical techniques to the distal limb and works by deep vein drainage of the lymphatic fluid. Lymphaticovenous anastomoses are best for lymphoedema of the upper limb, with less applicability for the lower limb. The supraclavicular lymph node flap can also be used for transfer. Combinations of lymph node transfer + modified Charles procedures are sometimes required for the cases with the worst fibrosis. Preservation of the deep fascia, prior to grafting, and control of infection are important principles. The Charles procedure should be avoided for the upper limb.

References

1. Jones B, Lo S. How long does a face lift last? Objective and subjective measurements over a 5-year period. Plast Reconstr Surg. 2012;130(6):1317–27.
2. Hodgkinson D. Five-year experience with modified Fogli/Lore's fascia fixation Platysmaplasty. Aesthet Plast Surg. 2012;36:28–40. https://doi.org/10.1007/s00266-011-9772-2.
3. Richardson W, Carman JB. On the fabric of the human body. Book 11, chapter XIII. Novatop, CA: Norman Publishing; 2009. p. 167–9. (English translation of Vesalius, A; De humani corporis fabrica, 1543 Bale).
4. Bensimon RH. Croton Oil Peels. Aesthet Surg J. 2008;28(1):1–14.

General Principles

4

Principles Are the Bedrock of Plastic Surgery and a
Starting Point for Constructing Sensible and Logical
Answers

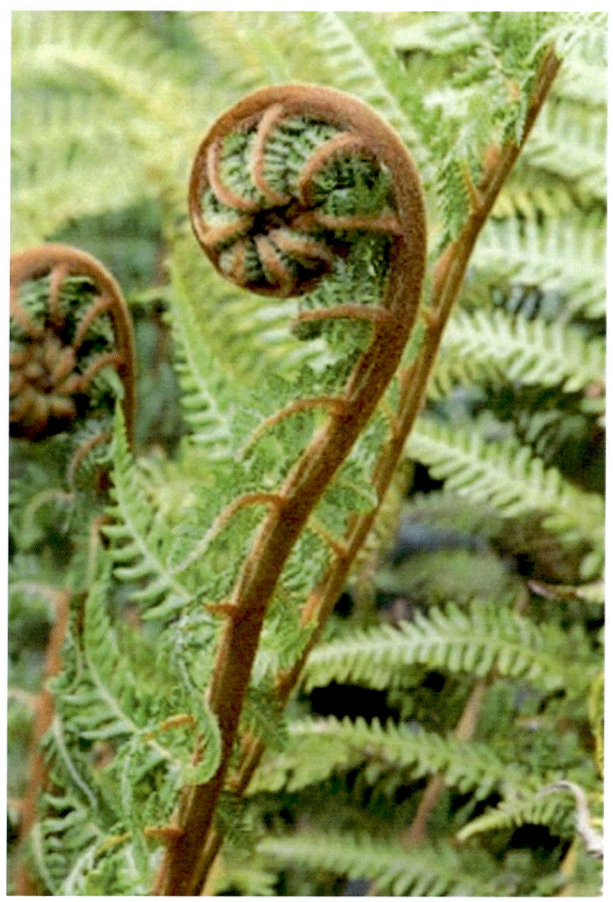

Koru

© Springer Nature Singapore Pte Ltd. 2018
M. F. Klaassen and E. Brown, *An Examiner's Guide to Professional
Plastic Surgery Exams*, https://doi.org/10.1007/978-981-13-0689-1_4

The Koru is a spiral shape, based on the shape of a new unfurling silver fern frond. In Maori culture it symbolises new life or beginnings, growth, strength regeneration and peace.

> *In plastic surgery, perfection is only just good enough.*
> *(Sir William M. Manchester, 1960s)*

4.1   Looking Back

The specialty of Plastic Surgery has a long and rich history dating back to the ancient Sanskrit text, Susruta Samhita in the sixth century BCE. Throughout surgical history, the giants of our specialty were keen observers and had a great ability to succinctly record general principles. Regardless of the problem, whether it be congenital or acquired, the plastic surgeon's task is to restore form, function and appearance. This can only be achieved by adapting one's knowledge of anatomy, physiology and wound healing to address reconstructive and aesthetic challenges. The use of general principles makes it possible for the plastic surgeon to devise creative solutions to an ever-increasing variety and complexity of problems that modern civilisation produces. Time will pass and generations of plastic surgeons will come and go, but the principles of plastic surgery will stand the test of time.

4.2   What Are Principles?

Principles are the fundamental underlying truths and beliefs that form the foundation of our knowledge and values and guide our actions. Everything can be reduced to a set of principles, rules or guidelines. In the surgical context, a principle is a basic guideline or common sense rule that we use intuitively in everyday practice to treat our patients. When we list the published general principles of Plastic Surgery, one cannot be surprised at how similar these are between authors.

Dr. Robert Chase (a leading plastic surgeon at Stanford University, California) noted that: A principle develops through a period of gestation, it is not born fully developed. Once born, a principle continues to evolve and to become more refined as new developments prompt expansion or modification of the principle. In rare instances, dramatic medical advances prompt expansion or modification of the principle. Unlike a technique, which ought to be replaced or refined regularly as new methods develop, the core of a principle is likely to survive [1] (Fig. 4.1).

We believe that by embracing basic reconstructive principles, the Plastic surgeon is equipped to be creative and innovative in seeking surgical solutions to complex problems. This enables us to create modifications to standard procedures to fit the surgical problem (and not make the problem fit a standard procedure).

In this chapter we will discuss General Principles which can be used for all aspects of Plastic and Reconstructive Surgery.

Fig. 4.1 Dr. Robert Chase of Stanford University, California

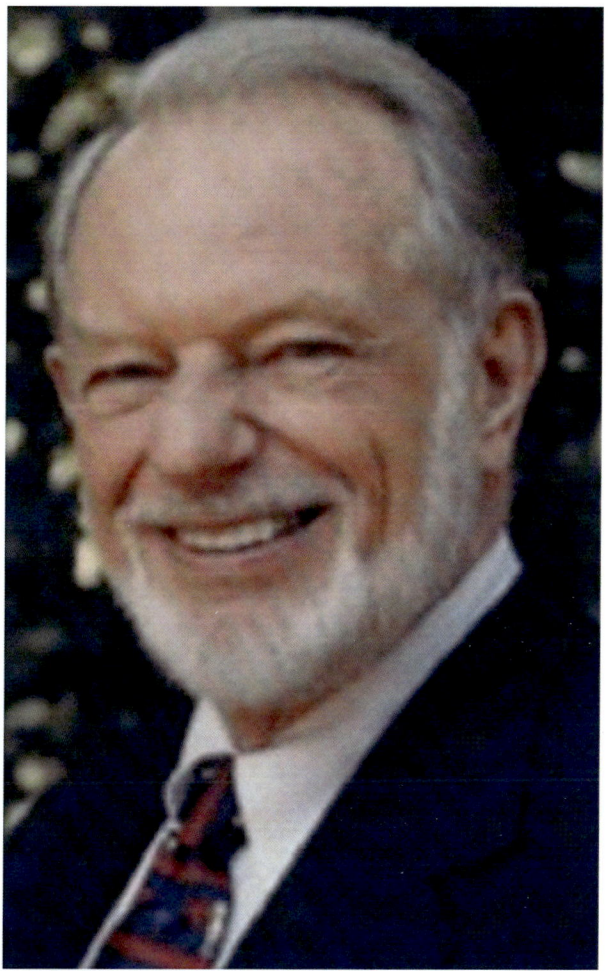

Some of these basic principles have changed very little since their enunciation centuries ago.

Let us start in the sixteenth century.

4.2.1 Ambrose Paré (French Barber Surgeon 1510–1590)
   (Fig. 4.2)

In 1564 Paré, by then with considerable surgical experience, quoted Celsus (75 BC to 50 AD)

> 'Wherefore you should cut off as little of that which is sound as you possibly can, yet so that you cut away that which is quicker, than leave behind anything that is perished.'

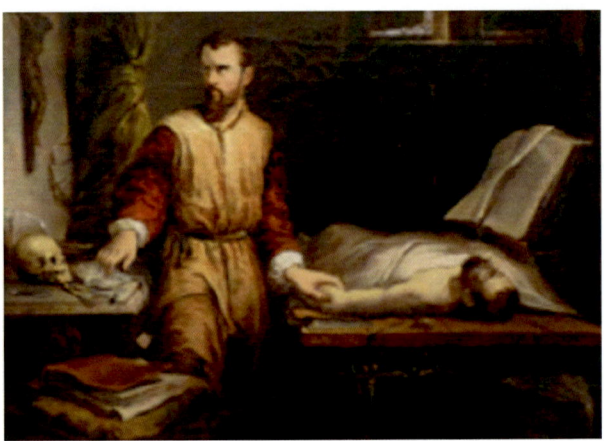

Fig. 4.2 Surgeon
Ambrose Paré

1. To take away what is superfluous. *To eliminate that which serves no purpose.*
2. To restore to their places things which are displaced. *This required recognition of normal parts and diagnosis of the abnormal position.*
3. To separate tissues which are joined together. *Separation of congenital syndactyly or acquired fusion due to burns.*
4. To join those tissues which are separate. *These required the ability to conceptualise the norm.*
5. To supply the defects of Nature. *Requires the ability to visualise restoration to a normal state.*

4.2.2 Gaspare Tagliocozzi (Italian Surgeon from Bologna 1545–1599) (Fig. 4.3)

In 1597 towards the end of his short life Tagliacozzi from Bologna, Italy recorded:

> We restore, repair and make whole those parts…..
> Which nature has given but which fortune has taken away,
> Not so much that they may delight the eye
> But that they may buoy up the spirit and
> Help the mind of the afflicted [2].

4.2.3 William Stewart Halsted (Johns Hopkins Hospital Founding Surgeon 1852–1922) (Fig. 4.4)

William Halsted promoted seven principles of wound care, known as the *Tenets of Halstead* in the 1890s. Whilst these were written for all surgeons, they are still very applicable to Plastic and Reconstructive Surgery this century.

Fig. 4.3 The Italian Renaissance surgeon Gaspare Tagliacozzi

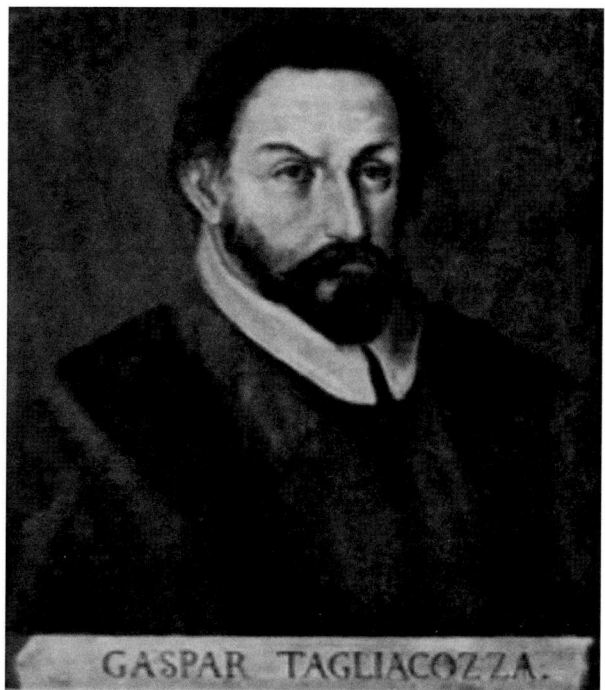

1. *Handle tissues gently*
2. *Achieve meticulous haemostasis*
3. *Preserve vascularity*
4. *Ensure strict asepsis*
5. *Ensure good approximation of tissues*
6. *Close the wound without tension*
7. *Avoid dead space*

4.2.4 Captain and Later Sir Harold D. Gillies (1892–1960) (Fig. 4.5)

Gillies, with his huge experience treating facial injuries inflicted during World War 1 developed a set of Principles about 1920 [3].

Pre-operative

1. *Mistakes in diagnosis due to inadequate examination are perhaps the commonest cause of indifferent treatment.*
2. *In planning the restoration, function is the first consideration … and the best cosmetic results are, as a rule, only to be obtained where function has been restored.*

Fig. 4.4 Professor
William Halsted of
Baltimore

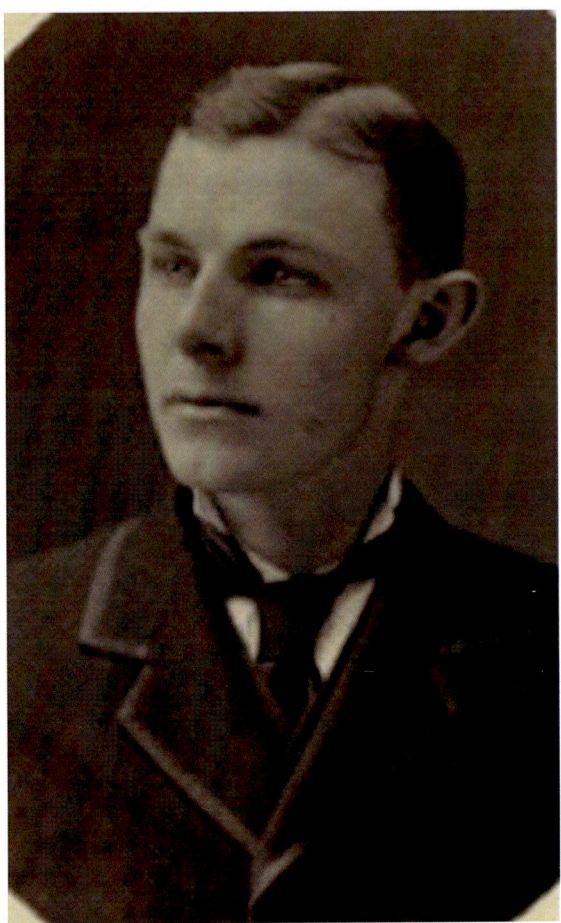

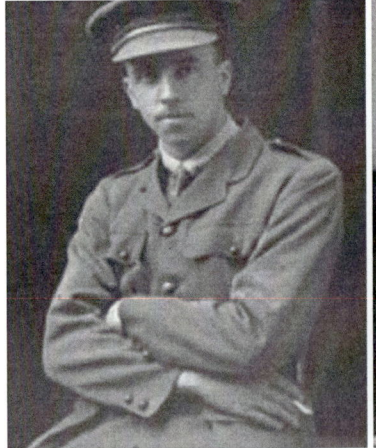 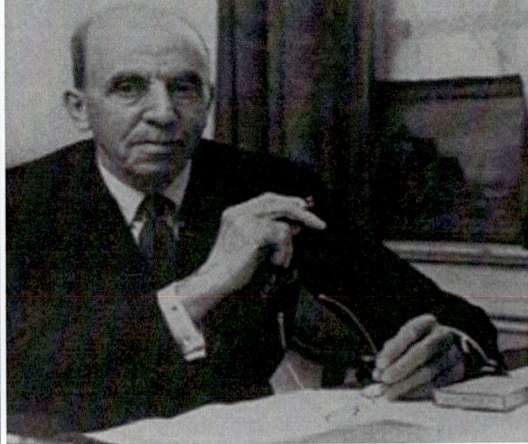

Fig. 4.5 Sir Harold Gillies the military and the civilian plastic surgeon

3. *The restoration is designed from within outwards. The lining membrane must be considered first, then the supporting structures, and finally the skin covering.*
4. *There is no royal road to the fashioning of the facial scaffold by artificial means: the surgeon must tread the hard and narrow way of pure surgery.*
5. *It may be laid down as a guiding maxim that the replacement should be as nearly as possible in terms of the tissues lost, i.e. bone for bone, cartilage for cartilage, fat for fat, etc.*

Intra-operative

1. *All normal tissue should be replaced as early as possible, and maintained in its normal position.*
2. *Speaking generally, the use of any foreign body is to be condemned whenever it is possible to substitute a graft from the patient himself. Any form of foreign body is a tissue irritant, and tends to give trouble early or late, in the attempt on the part of the tissues to remove it, whereas grafts, if successful in the early stages, continue satisfactorily.*
3. *The gain of skin below the mouth has to be written off against the loss, which occurs when the bed from which it was raised is closed.*
4. *Apart from those containing a definite artery such as the superficial temporal (the base of which may be cut quite narrow), the base should be at least as wide as any other part of the flap.*
5. *The pedicle is returned not earlier than 10 days in most cases, and it is of advantage largely to increase this interval where the blood supply of the receiving bed is dubious.*

Postoperative

1. *Disappointment is in store for him who would confine his repair to the surface tissues, heedless of Nature's lessons in architecture.*
2. *Satisfactory early results are obtained by very cautious and repeated injections of paraffin wax in small quantities, but the late results are rarely good and are often appalling this principle would be condemned in modern concepts.*
3. *For larger hollows, free fat and muscle grafts are used: these are naturally more uncertain of result … it is not yet established how they will be affected in conditions of wasting and in old age. The fat-graft however, owing to fat necrosis, often undergoes a partial absorption.*
4. *The production of an invisible scar is a question constantly exercising the mind of the plastic surgeon.*
5. *The factors necessary for the production of the optimum scar are: asepsis, avoidance of tension on the apposing sutures, perfect apposition of the skin edges, an often unknown personal factor in the patient, early removal of sutures.*

6. *The most frequent cause of failure of a Wolfe graft is lack of pressure firm enough to ensure complete apposition.*
7. *Time is the plastic surgeon's greatest ally, and at the same time his most trenchant critic.*

Gillies' 1920 principles were rewritten later to embrace his change from military to civilian plastic surgery, reduced in number and were known as *The Ten Commandments of Gillies.*

Gillies' ten commandments of plastic surgery

1. *Thou shalt make a plan.*
2. *Thou shalt have a style.*
3. *Honor that which is normal and return it to normal position.*
4. *Thou shalt not throw away a living thing.*
5. *Thou shalt not bear false witness against thy defect.*
6. *Thou shalt treat thy primary defect before worrying about the secondary one.*
7. *Thou shalt provide thyself with a lifeboat.*
8. *Thou shalt not do today what thou canst put off until tomorrow.*
9. *Thou shalt not have a routine*
10. *Thou shalt not covet thy neighbour's plastic unit, handmaidens, forehead flaps, Thiersch grafts, cartilage nor anything that is thy neighbour's*

These ten commandments were later increased to 16 Principles, by Gillies and Millard [4] (Fig. 4.6). In their chapter on Principles they stated that 'The father and mother of all principles in reconstructive surgery is that *plastic surgery is a constant battle between blood supply and beauty*'.

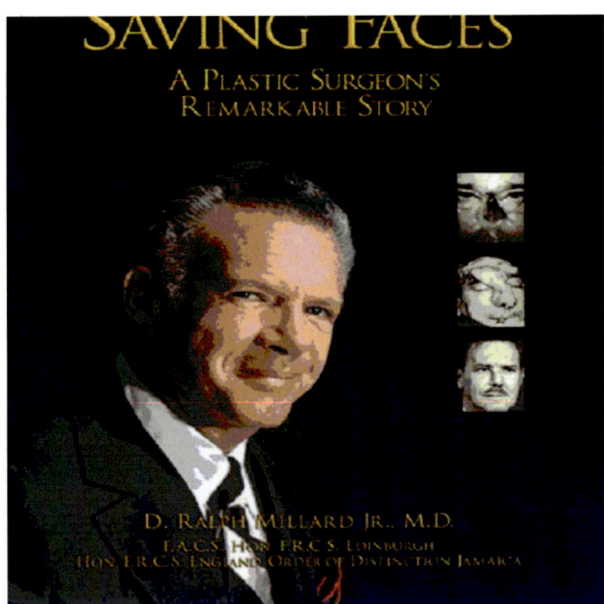

Fig. 4.6 Dr. D. Ralph Millard Jnr

1. *Observation is the basis of surgical diagnosis*
2. *Diagnose before you Treat*
3. *Make a plan and a pattern for this Plan.*
4. *Make a Record*
5. *The Lifeboat*
6. *A good style will get you through*
7. *Replace what is normal in normal position and retain it there*
8. *Treat the primary defect first*
9. *Losses must be replaced in kind*
10. *Do something positive*
11. *Never throw anything away*
12. *Never let routine methods become your master*
13. *Consult other specialists*
14. *Speed in surgery consists of not doing the same thing twice*
15. *The aftercare is as important as planning*
16. *Never do today what can honourably be put off till tomorrow.*

Dr. D. Ralph Millard (formerly a journalist before studying medicine) later expanded on these principles and classified them in to:

1. *Preparational* Principles
2. *Executional* Principles
3. *Innovational* Principles
4. *Contributional* Principles
5. *Inspirational* Principles

He promoted *The Plastic Surgeon's Creed* condensing the 33 principles to:

Know the ideal beautiful normal
Diagnose what is *present*, what is *diseased, destroyed, displaced, or distorted*, and what is in *excess*.
Then, guided by the normal in your mind's eye, utilise what you have to make what you *want*—and when possible *go for even better* than what would have been.

See Appendix B.

4.2.5 Sir William Manchester

(Trained in Plastic and Reconstructive surgery during World War 2 by Gillies, McIndoe and Mowlem) (Fig. 4.7).

Manchester had a huge influence on the Authors and constantly repeated his principles with almost religious fervour.

The Mantras of Manchester

- When faced with a plastic surgical Problem.
  - *Make an accurate diagnosis, taking in to account the patient's history.*

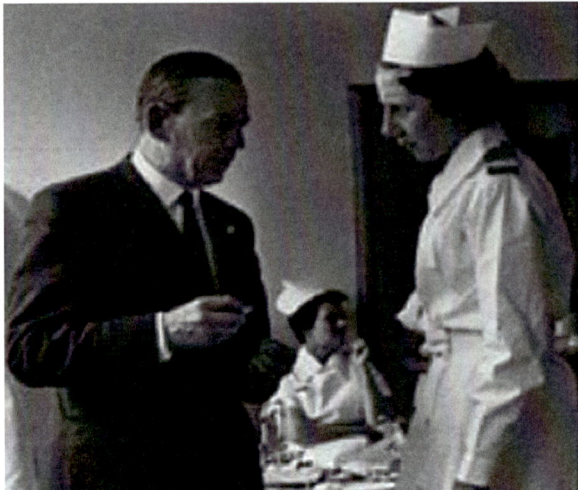

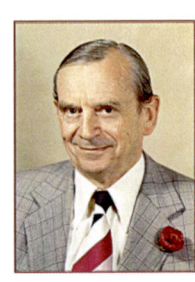

Sir William Manchester Oration

Fig. 4.7 Sir William M. Manchester and Sister 'Eddie' Edwards

- Is there any tissue missing or is it merely displaced?
- How much and of what tissue is missing or displaced?
  - *How much skin is missing?*
  - *How much subcutaneous tissue is missing?*
  - *How much muscle is missing?* etc.
- Review the methods available for reconstruction
  - *Can you repair it with local tissue?*
  - *Can you repair it with a free graft?*
  - *Can you repair it with a distant flap?*
  - *Can you repair it with a free flap?*
  - *A combination of any or all of the above.*

The result should be judged by the patient, and peers in the long-term follow-up clinic, that is, in "The Hall of Truth".

Always remember, "Perfection is only just good enough".

The authors have embraced the *16 Principles of Gillies and Millard* and the *Mantras of Manchester* in their practice over many years. In addition to these Principles we strongly recommend a further Principle, *Restoration of Function*.

4.2.6 How Does the Student of Plastic Surgery Use Principles in Surgical Practice?

During their training in Plastic and Reconstructive surgery, the trainee will be strongly influenced by the Principles espoused by their teachers and mentors [5–10].

Whilst each Principle is reduced to one line of text we believe that the trainee should have thought beyond these words to obtain the wider implications of that

Principle. In doing this, the Principle is enhanced and this will influence judgement and decision making and will lead to innovation in solving reconstructive problems. Sometimes the stated General Principles overlap with Specific Principles relating to Disciplines within Plastic Surgery. Robert Chase's Principle of using salvageable parts in severe hand injuries is a specific use of a Principle, compared with the general principle of Gillies and Millard, No. 9: *Losses must be replaced in kind.*

Let us take *Diagnosis of a skin tumour* as an example to study a Principle. This introduces your contact with the patient. Not only should you establish empathy with the patient, but *listen* to his or her concerns.

> Throughout the surgical period and long after it, the patient will lean heavily on the surgeon for mental support, for hope and encouragement ....
>
> *(Sir Archibald McIndoe 1958)*

During this initial patient contact you should be using your powers of *observation* where you can obtain much information about the patient and their problem. In general, does the patient look healthy? Note the site of the problem and mentally recall the local anatomy. This leads to the physical examination; looking at the tumour and its characteristics, the condition of the surrounding skin and noting various characteristics such as solar damage, laxity, relaxed skin tension lines and suitability for a local flap repair. Check out other areas which may be relevant to the diagnosis such as regional lymph nodes (this is also an opportunity to do a general skin check for other tumours and conditions). Additional tests such as tissue biopsy and radiology may be required to establish a diagnosis.

The diagnosis may or may not be immediately obvious. We recommend you look at the wider implications of your history and examination to make sure that nothing is missed.

If you cannot come up with a diagnosis consider the surgical sieve of medical school days.

Congenital, traumatic, neoplastic, inflammatory, etc.

Once you have made a diagnosis, consider the treatment. If it is a tumour, assess the consequences of its adequate excision.

How much tissue is missing? This is an opportunity to review the anatomy of the region and what and how much of each tissue has been excised.

The treatment plan involves a review of the methods of reconstruction of each missing tissue, repairing with like tissues.

- Primary closure
- Local flaps
- Free grafts
- Microvascular tissue transfer
- Pedicled flap transfer
- A combination of methods

When you have a plan, consider alternate treatment methods (a lifeboat) should the situation change during surgery.

Once the surgery is completed, consider post-operative management, including dressings and monitoring for flap vascularity.

A thoughtful appraisal of all the plastic surgery principles should give the exam candidate the tools to influence their judgement and decision making. Plastic surgery principles are the elementary truths which provide the framework for sound clinical and surgical practice. They are the quintessential structure of plastic surgery and the fabric of our plastic surgery tapestry. With them we can become good human tailors! Perhaps the most important principle for plastic surgeons is the eloquent dream of the late master plastic surgeon Dr. Madeleine Lejour [11] of Belgium, who in December 2007 wrote:

> I have a dream. I would like to see reconstructive and cosmetic surgery practiced only by well-trained surgeons, with high ethical standards, concerned with the service to their patients more than with money and self-promotion. If we could reach the high standards of my dream, there is no doubt that plastic surgery would progress much faster, and fewer patients would suffer from trial and error. I have that dream, and it will be my last professional contribution.

References

1. Chase RA. Belaboring a principle. Ann Plast Surg. 1983;11(3):255–60.
2. Burget GC, Menick FJ. Aesthetic reconstruction of the nose. St. Louis: Mosby; 1994.
3. Gillies HD. Plastic surgery of the face. London: Henry Froude, Hodder and Stoughton; 1920.
4. Gillies HD, Millard DR Jr. The principles and art of plastic surgery. Boston: Little, Brown; 1957.
5. Rana RE, Puri VA, Baliarsing AS. Principles of plastic surgery revisited. Indian J Plast Surg. 2004;37(2):124.
6. Millard DR. Principlization of plastic surgery. Boston: Little, Brown and Company; 1986.
7. Freshwater MF. A critical comparison of Davis' principles of plastic surgery with Gillies' plastic surgery of the face. J Plast Reconstr Aesthet Surg. 2011;64:17–26.
8. Pettit JA. Underlying principles of plastic surgery. Calif State J Med. 1922;20(11):398.
9. DeMichele T. The importance of principles-fact/myth. Posted February 7, 2017.
10. Mulliken JB, Martinez-Perez D. The principle of rotation advancement for repair of unilateral complete cleft lip and nasal deformity: technical variations and analysis of results. Plast Reconstr Surg. 1999;104:1247–60.
11. Lejour M. Looking back at 50 years of plastic surgery. Plast Reconstr Surg. 2007;120(7):2106–9. https://doi.org/10.1097/01.prs.0000287388.25651.65.

The Art of Writing Exam Answers

5

How to Become a Good Wordsmith so that Your Written Essays, Short Answers and Notes Are Precise, Relevant and Clear to the Reader

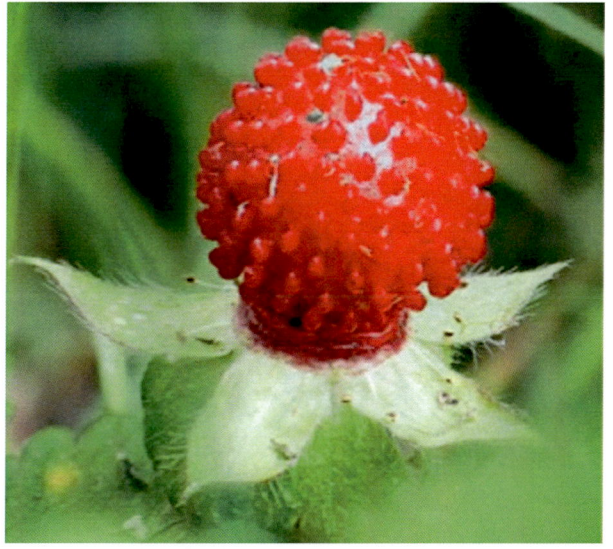

Potentilla indica

Writing is its own reward.

(Henry Miller)

5.1 Key Tips

1. Answer all questions
2. Write in a legible style (The RACS Court of Examiners is about to introduce TYPED answers, as the new standard)

© Springer Nature Singapore Pte Ltd. 2018
M. F. Klaassen and E. Brown, *An Examiner's Guide to Professional Plastic Surgery Exams*, https://doi.org/10.1007/978-981-13-0689-1_5

3. Consider the time allowed for each part of the question—this tells you how much is expected on that topic
4. Draw a diagram only if asked—any mistake would be more obvious

Certain aspects of professional exams in plastic surgery require a level of writing skill that conveys your clinical and scientific thinking. The ability to write concise and accurate answers to written questions is important for exam success. Your written word conveys to the examiner(s) reading it an indication of your thinking as a consultant plastic surgeon, your ability to interpret and understand the topic of the question and how you organise this into a communication that displays common-sense, consideration of the variables and focused patient care. In general terms and perhaps the key to writing competency is clear, logical and selective use of words. The less you write ensures that the reader will be engaged. More is less.

It is always a good idea to construct a plan or an overview for your written response. Over the many years of marking actual or mock written answers, I have observed how a clear and well-organised plan at the beginning heralds a good answer; an answer that is clearly a pass mark. The plan can be in any form including bullet points, headlines or an algorithm-like plan.

As *an example* a question about the management of a patient with inverted nipples would commence with:

Definition of inverted nipple and a classification for the different grades of inversion.
Aetiology and differential diagnosis.
Functional versus aesthetic concerns.
The context of inverted nipples – congenital, acquired or secondary to underlying pathology.
Management options – non-surgical versus surgical.
Your method of choice.
Technique.
Complications.
Patient issues.

A young woman with congenital inversion of her nipples is contrasted with a middle-aged woman who presents with unilateral inversion associated with pain, nipple discharge or nipple bleeding. The first scenario involves a stronger aesthetic, body image and self-confidence set of concerns, whilst the second raises the definite possibility of intraductal carcinoma. The history and examination of both cases requires a comprehensive consideration of the real risk of breast cancer and if this is real then further investigation with breast mammography, high-resolution ultrasound and MRI scanning should be suggested.

For the simple case of congenital nipple inversion, the consideration of management should include the issues of nipple hygiene, recurrent infections and the future of lactation potential with or without surgical correction.

Many different methods of surgical correction have been described. The most reliable is probably that described by Professor Neven Olivari of Cologne, where a small incision is made at the base of the inverted nipple, a skin hook is used to retract the inverted nipple and all the shortened nipple ducts are sharply released [1]. The resulting soft tissue gap is then closed with a buried purse-string suture. This method is simple, reproducible and reliable. The resulting scars are minimal and the surgery can be performed as an outpatient under local anaesthesia. Future breast feeding is unlikely, but Olivari's published series mentions a small percentage of patients who went on to successfully breast feed their babies. Spontaneous recanalisation is the likely reason in these rare cases. Other methods have been described using microscopic dissection of the nipple to preserve lactation function and various buried areolar flaps designed to support the everted nipple structure. These involve more soft tissue dissection, scarring and complications. The fundamental question is whether or not patients with inverted nipples will ever truly successfully breast feed with or without surgical correction. There has been a growing body of lactation specialist nurses who would argue otherwise but the reality is open to debate.

5.2   Types of Written Questions

1. Multiple choice
2. Short answers
3. Essays

Multiple choice questions are more the trend for the Part 1 FRACS exams. They are a feature of professional anaesthetic exams Part 2, FANZCA. The Part 2 or Final Fellowship exams for FRACS tend to be in a combination of short answer and long answer/essay form. The two written papers that candidates present for about a month before the oral examinations are usually 2 hours long. The questions are carefully constructed by members of the plastic surgery mini-court, several months before and will have indicators for how much time should be allocated by the writer.

5.3   Style of Written Questions

1. Knowledge style; assess the question and decide what knowledge needs to be conveyed: anatomical, pathological, clinical or diagnostic
2. Interpreting a particular clinical context with mature judgement and safe decision-making
3. Contrasting and comparing different approaches to the same clinical problem
4. Situation awareness, risk management
5. Problem solving

5.4   Feedback from 8 Years of Marking Mock (Practice) Written Questions

From a review of the data that we have recorded from successive coaching courses (2012–2018) for groups of presenting candidates, without identifying any of these young surgeons, prognostic indicators have been observed. From a total of 469 mock written responses the overall pass rate has been 60%. The set-up for the Mock Written Questions is this: candidates enrolled for our coaching courses are emailed the mock written questions, one at a time. They are instructed to set aside protected time to complete the answer, in usually 30 or 60 minutes.

Candidates practising the mock written questions in an exam context show a definite improvement in their success rate with practice and constructive feedback. Fifty seven percent of candidates completed 50% of the set mock written questions. The answers are marked with a purposefully high scholarly expectation within 24 hours of them being returned by email. Those candidates who fail or have only a marginal pass receive written feedback with constructive advice on how to improve their answers.

A small percentage of candidates completely misread the question or misdiagnose the clinical case in the question. This was in reference to the difference between the syndromes of hemifacial microsomia and hemifacial atrophy. An obvious disadvantage for some candidates is regurgitating a preconceived answer, which bears little relevance to the question asked. Another glaring fault was the failure to construct a plan at the beginning of the answer. Time management is also a challenge and candidates must learn to allocate enough time to segments of their answer, so that major omissions of knowledge and interpretation are minimised.

A real but occasional problem, given that handwritten answers are still the standard for the RACS final fellowship exams is illegible writing. Some candidates do struggle with this handicap even when counselled about it. The stress of the exam environment does not help this characteristic of illegibility, but it is a fundamental principle that the examinee must construct text and written language that can be read. Philip Carson FRACS, current Chairman of the RACS Court of Examiners revealed at the May 2018 ASC Education Session, that a move to TYPED answers is imminent.

Some other general guidelines for successful exam writing include the following:

1. Practice answering written questions under pressure, so that you become used to the 'test anxiety' reality of professional exams.
2. Develop time-use strategies, again under pressure with practice of mock written questions, until your writing skills improve.
3. Avoid guessing an answer, use deductive reasoning and commonsense based on first principles.
4. Don't try and bluff your answer.
5. Use key words that have clear meaning.

5.5   Previous Mock (Practice) Written Questions

Here are some examples of either real questions from past exams or mock questions designed for our coaching course for FRACS (Plastic & Reconstructive Surgery). *Model answers can be found in Appendix A at the end of the book.*

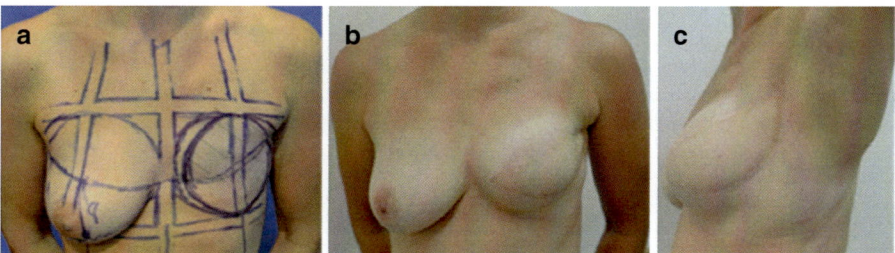

Fig. 5.1 (a–c) Images of 32-year-old left breast reconstruction case

5.5.1   Mock (Practice) 01 (Fig. 5.1)

A 32-year-old marine biologist is 2 years post left mastectomy for extensive DCIS with foci of invasion. She is nulliparous and has moderate ptosis of her contralateral right breast. After staged reconstruction of a left breast mound with tissue expander covered with a latissimus dorsi myocutaneous flap and definitive matched anatomical permanent submuscular implant **she is very content with her appearance in clothing and declines further surgery including nipple-areola reconstruction and right mastopexy to give her perfect breast symmetry.** *Discuss (30 min).*

5.5.2   Mock (Practice) 02

For cutaneous defects of the face post skin cancer excision, a number of repair techniques are available including healing by secondary intention, direct closure, local flaps and skin grafts. Consider different regions of the face, the type of skin cancer prevalent to each and discuss your preferred repair method (60 min).

5.5.3   Mock (Practice) 03

Consider the management of hand fractures, mechanism of injury and methods available for successful outcomes functionally and rehabilitatively (60 min).

5.5.4   Mock (Practice) 04 (Fig. 5.2)

A 57-year-old woman presents with an infiltrating ulcerated BCC of her right conchal fossa. She is aware of ageing changes in her lower face. Discuss a management plan that addresses both the skin cancer and her ageing concerns (60 min).

Fig. 5.2 (**a, b**) 57-year-old woman with infiltrating BCC of right conchal fossa and lower facial ageing stigmata

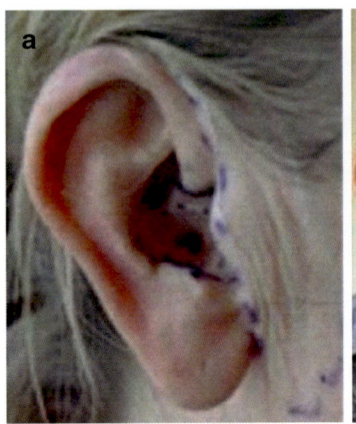 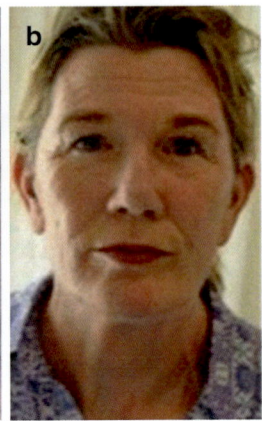

5.5.5   Mock (Practice) 05

Compare and contrast the surgical techniques for rhinoplasty including open versus closed techniques and septoplasty (60 min).

5.5.6   Mock (Practice) 06

Outline the theory and practice of neonatal ear moulding for auricular deformations (30 min).

5.5.7   Mock (Practice) 07 (Fig. 5.3)

This 20-year-old student suffers from Ehlers-Danlos syndrome and has had previous bilateral first rib resections for thoracic outlet syndrome. She is on significant analgesic medications for chronic pain secondary to her joint instabilities which involve her shoulders and her vertebral column. She requests a bilateral breast reduction for her pendulous breast hypertrophy. Discuss your management strategies including perioperative risk factors (60 min).

5.5.8   Mock (Practice) 08 (Fig. 5.4)

This fit 45-year-old woman requests restoration of breast volume and projection. She is not keen on breast implants and just wants to have a more feminine appearance. Describe the conversation you would have with her and what your recommendation would be. Justify your decision for management (60 min).

Fig. 5.3 20-year-old woman with Ehlers-Danlos Syndrome and severe grade III bilateral breast ptosis

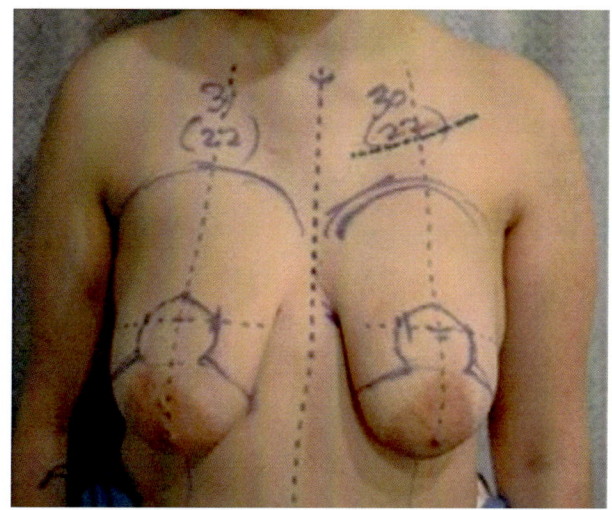

Fig. 5.4 This 45-year-old woman has post-partum breast involution and requests advice about restoration of her breast volume and projection

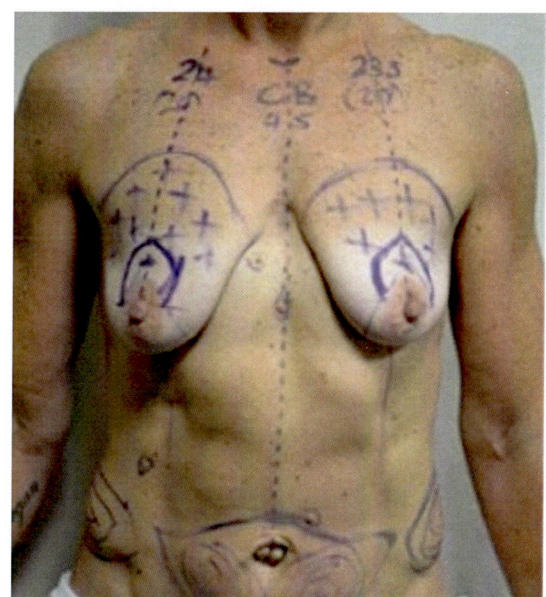

Reference

1. Olivari N. Practical plastic and reconstructive surgery: an atlas of operations and techniques. Heidelberg: Kaden; 2008. ISBN-10: 3922777848.

Long Clinical Cases

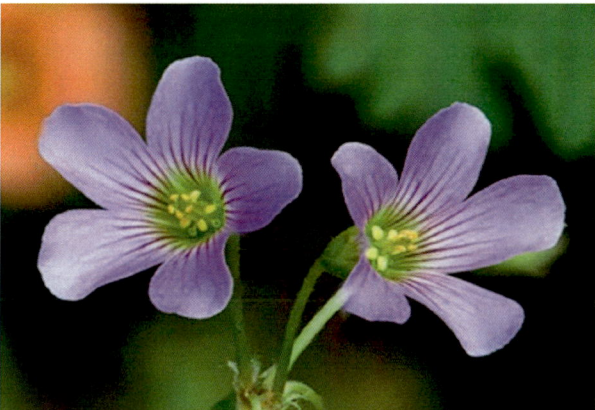

Oxalis debilis

The good physician treats the disease; the great physician treats the patient who has the disease.

(William Osler)

6.1   Key Tips

1. The examiners allow you 10 minutes for taking history and examination—make full use of this time
2. Some direct questioning may be required in the history
3. Respect the patient's privacy and comfort during your clinical examination. Avoid painful areas

© Springer Nature Singapore Pte Ltd. 2018
M. F. Klaassen and E. Brown, *An Examiner's Guide to Professional Plastic Surgery Exams*, https://doi.org/10.1007/978-981-13-0689-1_6

4. Present your findings according to a logical format: history, examination, investigation, provisional diagnosis, your preferred treatment plan and if time allows, other options
5. Treatment is not just an operation—consider the whole patient
6. If required ask permission to write things down as you go

Long cases are generally those where the candidate spends 10 minutes taking a history, performing a physical examination, making a diagnosis and deciding on a management plan. The diagnosis and management plan are discussed with the two examiners in the remaining 20 minutes. The examiners will have a discussion with the candidate during this time and ask a number of case-related questions. The candidate will usually see two long cases in succession and in the FRACS exam for plastic surgery, a pass mark for both cases is mandatory.

There are some general guidelines for the performance expected in the long case clinical exams. Sometimes the candidate may be presented with a short referral letter introducing the case. The long cases and the short cases are probably the most stressful components of the exam and it goes without saying that the candidate should be both physically and mentally well prepared. It is important to avoid any reference to the examiners or personal discussion. Answer the questions directly and briefly and don't ever try to 'bluff' your way through a response, as this will be obvious. There are some behaviour patterns during the exam which are best avoided: unnecessary reference to the literature will not impress, flattery will get you nowhere, avoid lengthy verbose answers and rapid, aggressive talking.

The commonly presenting long cases may be paediatric or adult and involve conditions such as cleft lip and palate, breast reconstruction, breast reduction, facial tumour, facial palsy, major burn scars, brachial plexus injury, congenital hand anomaly, chronic osteomyelitis, chronic radiation injury, facelift and body contouring problems.

The context of this examination is akin to seeing a new patient in an outpatient clinic with two witnesses who then test your evaluation of the case. *After 10 minutes* of history and examination the candidate should move quickly to summarise the case, offer a differential diagnosis and overview of their management plan. The summary should be comprehensive but precise. It should include age and occupation of the patient, relevant past medical history, family history, drug and allergic history and the dominant physical signs. There may be radiological images or blood results available for interpretation. In summarising the clinical problem or diagnosis, technical language can be helpful to present a clear picture (Fig. 6.1).

Example: this 49-year-old medical secretary was concerned about the loose skin of her lower face and neck.

The key features of concern for her are: deepening nasolabial folds, asymmetrical platysma bands in her anterior neck, submental fullness and obliteration of the youthful cervicomental angle on the profile view.

After summarising your findings a management plan is presented. This should include possible problems and risk factors, the timing of treatment and the expected outcome.

The examiners will then lead the conversation with a series of specific questions of a technical and clinical management nature.

Fig. 6.1 49-year-old medical secretary concerned about the development of lower face and neck laxity

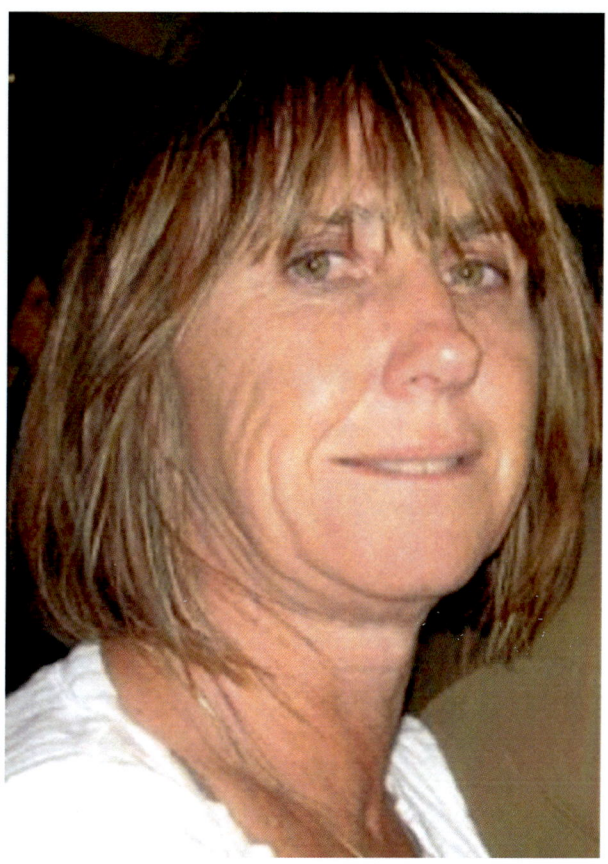

Let us now consider some common examples of Long Cases and strategies on how to perform well.

6.2   Breast Reconstruction

Example: Six months ago this 49-year-old woman had a complete mastectomy for a grade 2 invasive ductal carcinoma of the left breast. A sentinel node biopsy was negative, her oestrogen receptor status positive, and she was on Tamoxifen medication. She had a relatively high Body Mass Index (BMI). She underwent a staged breast reconstruction and Fig.6.2b shows the result after the first stage, following a moderate right breast reduction mammoplasty and a surgical 'delay' of the deep epigastric vascular pedicles for a proposed TRAM flap reconstruction.

This is a common exam scenario. You need to be efficient in your history taking and physical examination (10 minutes of the 30 minutes allowed), and be prepared to present a comprehensive and sensible summary of the long case for further questioning and discussion over the remaining 15–20 minutes. This summary should demonstrate your prioritising and organisational skills in planning a course of management for this patient.

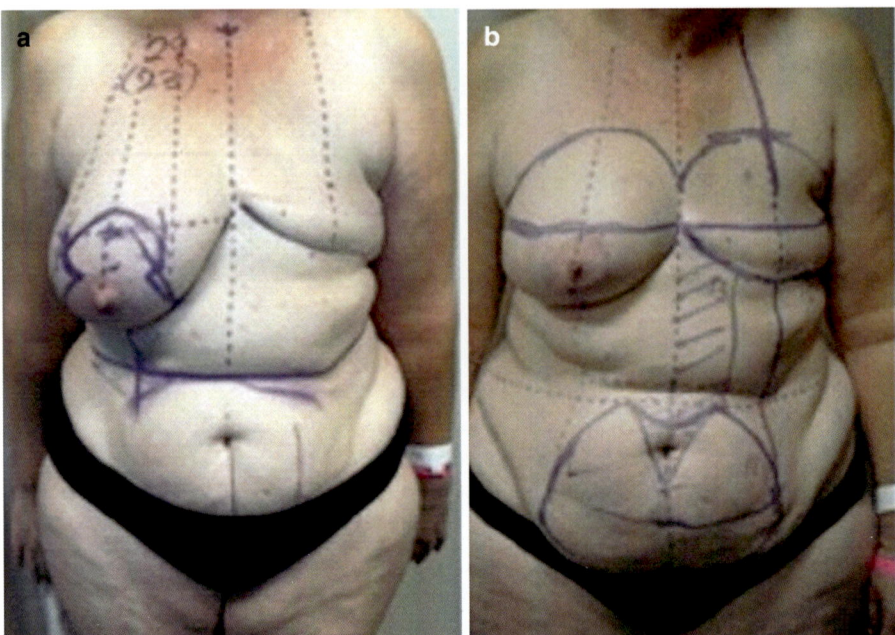

Fig. 6.2 (**a**) 49-year-old woman post left mastectomy for cancer. (**b**) same patient following contralateral breast reduction and surgical delay of a pedicled TRAM flap

Other aspects of management will include timing of the procedure, anaesthesia, post-operative management and monitoring, potential complications, the role of radiotherapy and prophylactic mastectomy for the opposite breast in high risk patients.

The discussion with the two examiners would then develop down a number of potential pathways including: the incidence and aetiology of breast cancer, options for her breast reconstruction and timing, prosthetic versus non-prosthetic options (external and implanted), risk factors for local recurrence, disseminated metastases, non-synchronous breast cancer in her contralateral breast, genetic risk factors, technical factors relating to flap anatomy, free tissue transfer versus pedicle flap alternatives, advantages, disadvantages and personal preferences. Other avenues of enquiry could include: potential complications and their management including flap and flap donor site complications such as necrosis (partial or complete), fat necrosis and infection, delayed healing, abdominal weakness and abdominal herniae, morphological changes in flap form with time, and the influences of adjuvant radiation therapy and chemotherapy. Timing of breast reconstruction whether immediate or delayed, the role of prophylactic mastectomy for high risk patients with familial genetic risk BRACA genes 1 & 2 and anaesthetic and perioperative management issues are common discussion points.

6.3   **Skin Cancers of the Face** (Fig. 6.3)

Example: This 81-year-old woman presented with two BCCs on her upper left face, one just lateral to the left periorbital margin, 3 cm in diameter and the other close to the upper pre-auricular region and 2 cm in diameter.

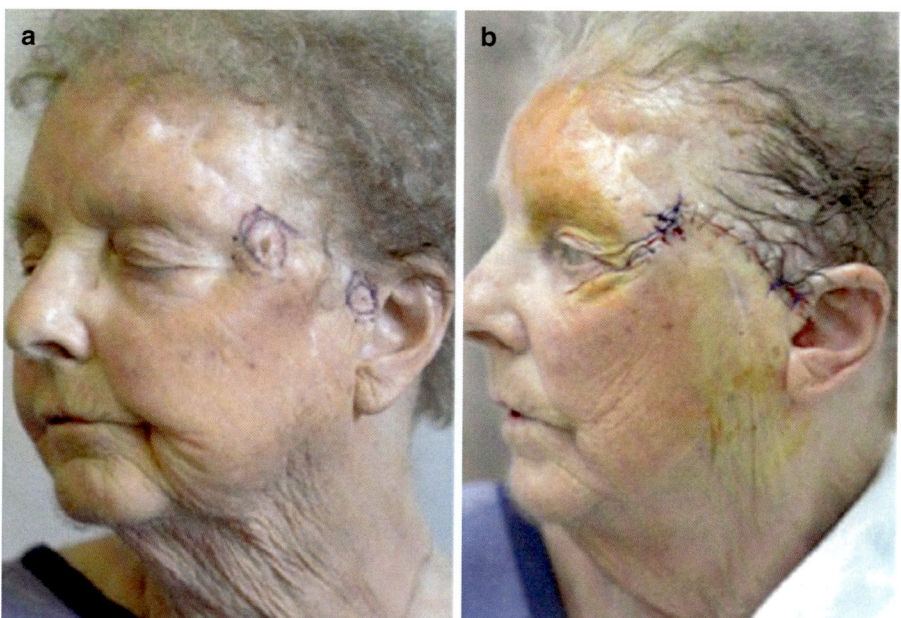

Fig. 6.3 (**a**) 81-year-old patient with infiltrating basal cell carcinomata left temple and left preauricular region. (**b**) Same patient following wide excision of both BCCs and repair with a Flicklift advancement flap

Three years ago she had an SCC widely excised from her left forehead and a local H-plasty flap repair. Healing of this repair was delayed by her immunosuppressive medication (Methotrexate) for chronic rheumatoid arthritis and a Clostridium difficile septicaemia, necessitating hospital admission.

Local examination revealed the two BCCs, scarring on the forehead following previous surgery and skin laxity of her lower face and neck.

The various repair options resulting from wide excision of the tumours were considered and included local flaps, full thickness skin grafts and a flap to utilise the spare skin of the lower face and neck.

My choice after careful discussion with the patient was the use of a broad, inferiorly based left facelift flap, designed over the SMAS layer and combining the Anterior Flick Lift to support the repair. The Flicklift is a minimalist aesthetic rejuvenation method for the ageing face developed by Levick and Frame from England, utilising a limited SMAS flap which is anchored by a strong figure-of-8, nonabsorbable suture to the deep temporal fascia. The SMAS flap in this reconstructive application (coined Aesthetica) supports the elderly thin advancement cheek flap and preserves its perforator blood supply.

The discussion with the examiners would be fairly predictable and could include:

Solar damage to the skin (Ian McGregor used to talk about 'field change' indicating an area of obvious solar damage).

The various types of facial skin cancers in the elderly.

Different forms of BCC such as nodular, sclerosing/morphoeic, basi-squamous, peri-neural invasion and microinfiltration.

Surgical resection margins.

Preservation or sacrifice of important landmarks and the aesthetic reconstruction with either skin grafts or local flaps.

The concepts of CLEAR and DRAPE are a convenient direction, in which the candidate can lead the examiners. *DRAPE* is Felix Behan's *Delayed Reconstruction After Pathological Examination*, a modern application of the Mohs Micrographic Surgery concept and based on the much more oncologically sound technique of margin-controlled tumour excision. In this technique, tangential incomplete resection of the cancer is avoided. I have added *CLEAR*, which is *Complete Local Excision & Aesthetic Reconstruction*, which combines wide local excision and reconstruction that considers the relaxed skin tension lines and aesthetic anatomical subunits. Again this is a modern alternative to Mohs surgery. For completeness I have also added to the strategy *PACS*, which stands for *Proper Anaesthetic Care & Safety*. This defines the safe and efficacious use of local anaesthetic, with or without intravenous sedation, proper monitoring of the patient's vital signs and also the addition of the different forms of general anaesthesia in appropriate cases. There is more about PACS in Chap. 10.

6.4   Foot Reconstruction (Fig. 6.4)

Example: This 36-year-old woman sustained a compound degloving injury to the dorsolateral aspect of her right foot, when she was accidentally hit with the revolving metal blades of a concrete polishing machine.

She presented with chronic neuropathic pain, suggestive of a sural nerve neuroma, was unable to stand for any length of time due to pain and unable to continue her work as a Hairdresser.

Examination revealed hypertrophic scars on the dorsolateral side of the right foot, hypersensitivity to touch in this area, loss of active flexion of the fourth and fifth toes due to extensor tendon tethering and normal foot pulses. There was anaesthesia in the sural nerve distribution on her foot and her gait was considerably impaired by pain on weight-bearing. The injured right foot is compared with the

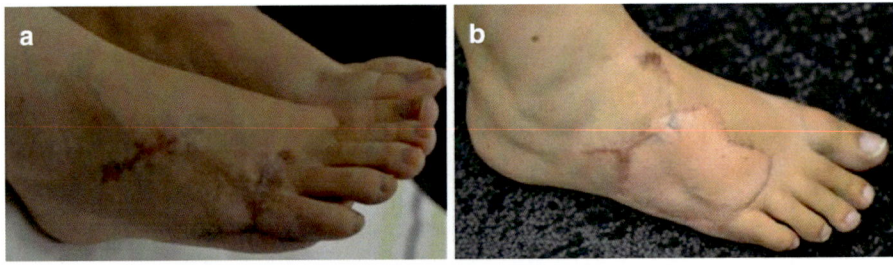

Fig. 6.4 (**a**) 36-year-old patient following concrete polisher trauma and degloving injury to the dorsum of her right foot. (**b**) Result of scar release, tenolysis and reconstruction of skin defect, with free radial forearm flap

normal left foot. A good candidate would consider measuring and comparing the circumferences of both feet.

Is there tissue missing? Yes.

Review of her Orthopaedic medical records indicate she had a degloving injury of soft tissues of the dorsum of the foot and a transverse fracture of the fifth metatarsal. The wound edges were debrided and the wounds repaired under tension. Some skin necrosis was noted following plaster cast removal. A recent plain X-ray confirmed that the metatarsal fracture was soundly united (Fig. 6.5).

Are there any local flaps that could make good the expected skin defect following release of the scars, extensor tenolysis and sural nerve neurolysis? No.

The wide zone of trauma and the scarcity of soft tissues confirm this. A distant flap is required and the choices would be between a free groin flap or a radial forearm flap. The groin flap has the most concealed donor site, but the pedicle of the superficial circumflex iliac artery is short.

Her groin skin was thickened with psoriasis and considered unsuitable for reconstruction of her foot. The non-dominant radial forearm donor site was the next best flap choice, with a long pedicle, thin pliable skin which would match the dorsal foot skin and the potential for vascularised tendon and nerve grafts if needed. The flap donor site could be closed with an ulnar-based transposition flap plus skin graft to the forearm defect. Later tissue expansion could be applied to improve the donor scar.

The patient is prepared for a long microvascular reconstructive operation. The procedure requires a two-surgeon team, expert anaesthetist and a nursing team familiar with the techniques of microvascular surgery. The operation is expected to take 6 hours and the patient will require 5–7 days in hospital and 3–4 months of rehabilitation. She is shown at 6 months post reconstruction (Fig. 6.4) with a normal gait and the only residual problem being some ongoing stiffness in her left wrist donor (Fig. 6.6).

Fig. 6.5 Plain X-Ray of right foot after degloving trauma

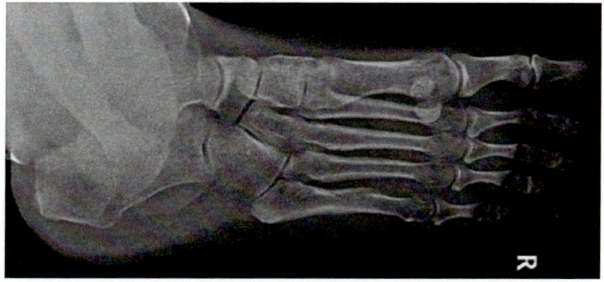

Fig. 6.6 Image of radial forearm flap donor site repaired with an ulnar-based flap

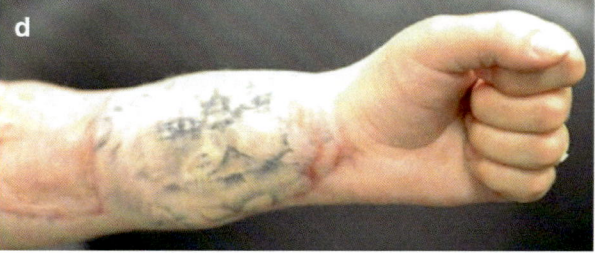

The discussion and questioning would focus on a number of clinical and technical principles:

The mechanism of injury and the contribution of the primary trauma management to the subsequent functional disability and suffering, the donor site selection process, the reconstruction of missing components—skin, gliding fascial tissue, extensor tendons and peripheral nerves. Microvascular surgical technique, teamwork, dual-surgeon approach for reducing operative time and efficiencies, post-operative flap monitoring, vascular flow problems at the microanastomoses and strategies to minimise this.

There was a very significant skin defect that had been underestimated by the primary orthopaedic trauma team. The importance of Interdisciplinary collaboration and support for complex limb trauma involving bone and soft tissue deficits is essential to optimise functional outcomes for the patients with severe lower limb trauma.

6.5   Facial Rejuvenation (Fig. 6.7)

This 59-year-old woman had an upper blepharoplasty 14 years previously and is now presenting for facial rejuvenation. She is conscious of atrophy, laxity and sagging of her mid face. She wants to look fresh and more youthful, but not in an unnatural way. On initial examination she has a round face with reasonable skin quality. There is some brow asymmetry with the left brow lower than the right and associated lateral upper lid hooding despite the previous upper blepharoplasty. She demonstrates some hollowing of the temples and infraorbital regions with flattening of the upper oblique cheek contour but minimal nasolabial folds. Her lower cheeks show good volume but there is early jowl formation and Marionette lines at her oral

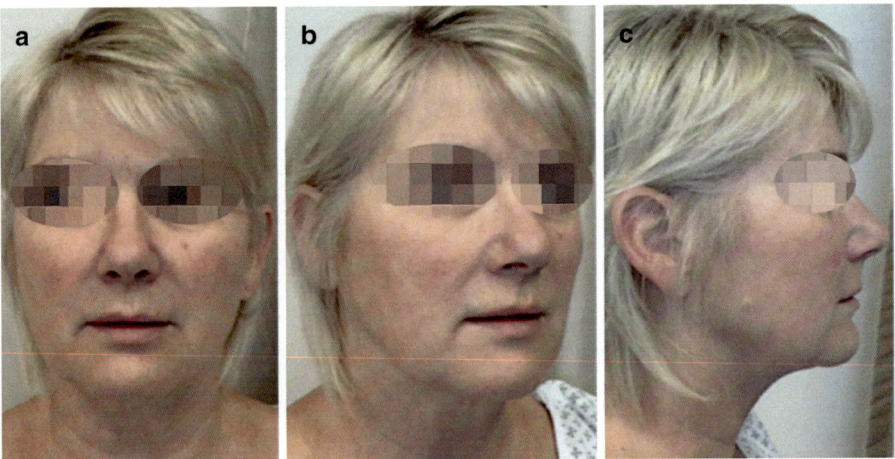

Fig. 6.7 (**a–c**) 59-year-old woman requests face and neck rejuvenation surgery. Previous successful upper blepharoplasty 14 years previously

commissures consistent with ageing. There are early platysmal bands anteriorly which appear symmetrical and some loss of the acute cervicomental angle of lateral view. Her neck is relatively short. Her nose is aesthetically pleasing with a straight dorsum, tip projection and an obtuse columellar-upper lip angle, again on the profile view. There is some loss of her upper lip volume with superficial vertical rhytids but preservation of her lower lip vermillion volume.

Methods of facial rejuvenation are many and are selected based on the patient's wishes and the surgeon's experience. All surgeons have been influenced by their mentors and adopt individual styles. For the exam candidate, with little experience in facial rejuvenative surgery it is important to concentrate on the anatomy of facial ageing and surgical principles to restore youthful appearances.

The good candidate should recognise and mention the obvious signs of aging in face and neck. Important anatomical points include: SMAS-Platysma structures and the associated retaining ligaments, Loré's fascia, fat pads and the junction zone between the anterior and lateral facial planes (major facial pilaster). Loré's fascia is a thickening of the parotid fascia in the pretragal region and also that fascia which descends down in front of the facial nerve and attaches to the styloid process + tympanic fissure. In reality it is a stout skull-based ligament with adequate strength to support the traction of the tissues in a permanent way. Dr. Darryl Hodgkinson emphasises this ligament in his modified Fogli approach to total neck rejuvenation [1].

The platysma muscles in the aged neck may display variable morphologies including laxity with skin wrinkling and laxity with platysma muscle spasm, known as platysmal bands. Dr. Daniel Labbé has recently described the additional laxity of the anterior bellies of digastric muscle, mylohyoid and the role of the cervico-mandibular subplatysmal ligament in ageing of the neck [2].

Pre-surgery assessment needs to determine which platysma bands need to be resected, which bands can be ignored and which bands can be retracted vertically and fixed to Loré's fascia. The submental incision is useful for access to the anterior bands, digastric muscles, submental, interplatysmal and subplatysmal fat pads. It is best to do this after the platysma muscle has been elevated and fixed vertically to the anchor point. Flaccid platysma bands are best resected. Unfurling of the horizontal wrinkles and tightening of the lower neck skin results in a 'tallness' of the neck. This is significant because a tall, well-toned neck is a sign of youth and beauty. The lower face and upper neck are addressed and access gained through limited incisions just inside the temporal hairline and extending down to the earlobe along the pretragal sulcus or post-tragal region as first described by Joseph [3].

The correcting vectors of lift should be vertical to counter the forces of gravity on the lax musculofascial layers. Upper fixation of the plication sutures on the SMAS-Platysma layers can be either to the periosteum of the zygomatic arch or to the deep temporal fascia. Once the excess skin is trimmed and wound closure achieved additional volume augmentation of the face can be achieved with judiciously placed autologous fat grafts. Post-operative care is important and Frame et al. [4] have described keeping the patients in a soft cervical collar for 2 weeks. The complications of face and neck lift surgery are important to note:

1. Haematoma requiring evacuation
2. Infection and skin necrosis
3. Seroma requiring aspiration
4. Temporary facial nerve weakness
5. Damage to the greater auricular nerve
6. Scar revision
7. Secondary or maintenance surgeries for persistent or recurrent laxity
8. Dissatisfied patients even after 6 months have passed

6.6   Amputation Stump Problems (Fig. 6.8)

*This 57-year-old former nurse sustained multiple injuries in a motor vehicle acci-
dent, when she was aged 19 years. Following several unsuccessful orthopaedic procedures, she required a high right above-knee amputation. Over several years this
has been a challenge for her with complex regional pain syndrome, phantom limb
pain and inability to wear a standard suction above-knee prosthesis. Prosthetic
rehabilitation with osseo-integrated technology had been considered but due to
logistical obstacles including funding, was not practical. She has extreme hypersensitivity of the end of her stump with a trigger point and a recent MRI scan confirms
a neuroma of the distal sciatic nerve. She can no longer live with the chronic pain
and various combinations of strong analgesic medications fail to give relief.
Surgical resection of the sciatic neuroma is indicated. This is best approached with
the patient prone, under general anaesthetic and with a high thigh tourniquet. The
nerve will be near the distal end of the stump and deep to the hamstring muscles.
After resecting the neuroma the choices will be to bury the end in either femoral
bone or hamstring muscles. The future prospects of osseo-integrated prosthetic*

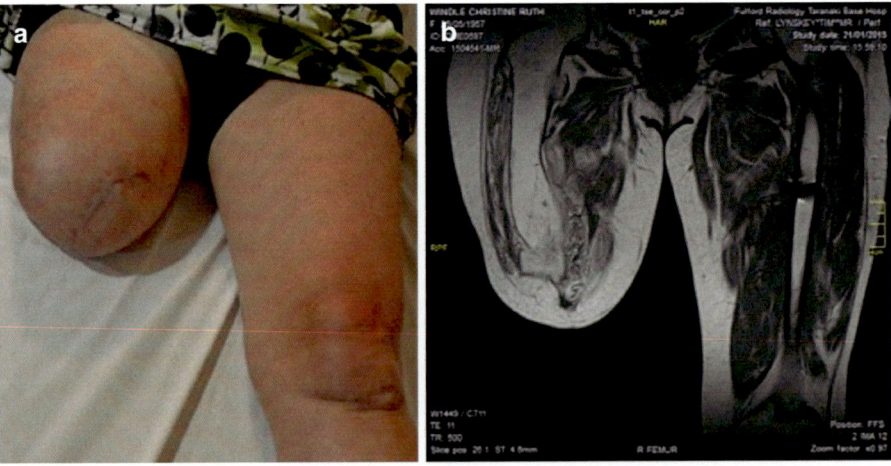

Fig. 6.8 57-year-old former nurse with longstanding post-traumatic Right above-knee amputation
stump, associated with chronic neuropathic pain and a neuroma of the sciatic nerve remnant

rehabilitation possibly preclude the bone site although this would be my preference for preventing recurrent neuroma. Perioperative analgesia will need careful planning given her chronic pain history and a patient-controlled-analgesia infusion would seem appropriate. I would liaise with her orthopaedic specialists although it would seem she has lost confidence in all of them. This is a difficult case and many careful discussions about the risks, potential complications and eventual outcome need to be had with the patient and her family.

This is a good long case with many aspects of trauma, secondary reconstruction, amputation stump problems and functional gait issues, rehabilitation, chronic neuropathic pain management and the role of pharmacology, transcutaneous nerve stimulation or surgery. It is also a case which highlights the importance of listening to and connecting with your patients. This was a principle so well demonstrated and applied by Sir Archibald McIndoe with his management of hundreds of burned aircrew in WWII.

References

1. Hodgkinson D. Total neck rejuvenation using a modified Fogli approach and selective resection of anterior platysmal bands. Clin Plast Surg. 2014;41:73–80.
2. Labbe D, Giot JP. Open neck contouring. Clin Plast Surg. 2014;41:57–63.
3. Joseph J. Cheekplasty (meloplasty). In: Rhinoplasty & facial plastic surgery with supplement on mammaplasty. Leipzig: Curt Kabitzsch Press; 1931. p. 621–8. (English translation by Stanley Milstein. Phoenix: Columella Press; 1987).
4. Frame JD, Frame JE. The concept of safer Facelifting. J Cosmet Dermatol. 2004;3:215–22.

Short Clinical Cases

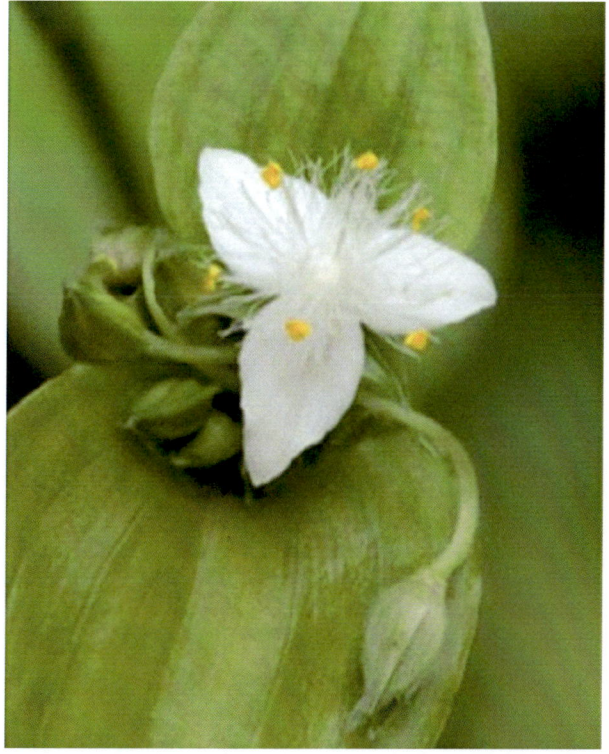

Tradescantia flumiensis

Observe, record, tabulate, communicate. Use your five senses.
(William Osler)

© Springer Nature Singapore Pte Ltd. 2018
M. F. Klaassen and E. Brown, *An Examiner's Guide to Professional
Plastic Surgery Exams*, https://doi.org/10.1007/978-981-13-0689-1_7

7.1   Key Tips

1. Listen to the question
2. Do a limited examination depending on the question

In the FRACS exam for plastic surgery the six or more short cases carry equal significance with the two long cases. As with the long cases, it is essential that you pass this segment of the exam.

Over approximately 30 minutes you will be lead around these short cases and the rules of engagement are: that you make a *spot diagnosis* and demonstrate any relevant clinical signs. The two examiners then take turns to ask you specific questions about the case, usually clinical questions but not excluding anatomical, pathological and management issues. Over the years the sample and type of short cases can be predicted with some confidence but the local hospital institutions providing the cases can add variation to this (adult versus paediatric cases). As with the long cases, keep your answers to the questions brief and precise. Correct use of terminology, classification systems, anatomical descriptors is helpful and recommended.

Here are some common examples of short cases and recurring themes for this segment of the exam:

7.2   Case 01

The left hand and right-dominant hand of a 48-year-old man, with Dupuytren's diathesis and a strong family history. He had a limited fasciectomy to the left hand 5 years ago and following recurrence, a radical dermo-fasciectomy 1 year ago (Fig. 7.1).

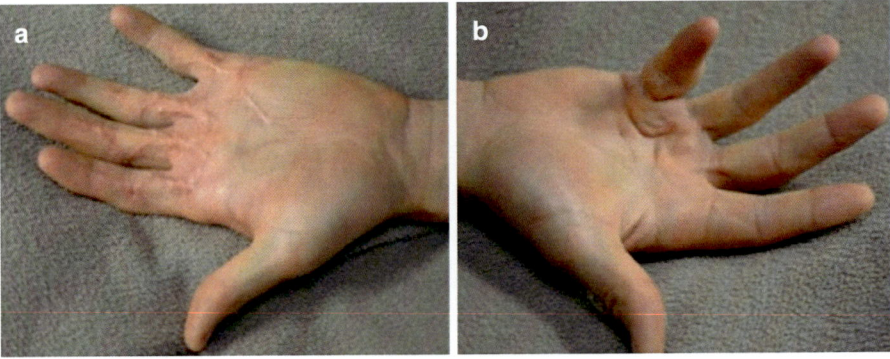

Fig. 7.1 (**a**) Left non-dominant hand of 48-year-old man, one year following radical fasciectomy for recurrent Dupuytren's contractures. (**b**) Right dominant hand of same man with recurrent flexion contractures of little, ring and middle fingers

This has given him reasonable left hand function but with hypertrophic scarring.

The dominant right hand has recurrent Dupuytren's nodules and bands to the little, ring and middle fingers with fixed flexion contractures and skin involvement to the MCPJ and PIPJ of the little finger.

The discussions and questions may cover:

Access incisions with Z-plasties, Bruner's zig-zag method, local keystone perforator flaps for skin defect closure, skin grafts, open-palm method of McCash, with secondary intention healing. Associated conditions with fibromatosis like Peyronie's (penis) and Ledderhose's (plantar fascia). Garrod's dorsal knuckle pads over the proximal inter-phalangeal finger joints, skin pits and indurated skin.

Aetiologies, diseased fibroblastic stem cells, risk factors, precise atraumatic dissection of the digital neurovascular bundles, limited versus radical fasciectomy, the role of fasciotomy and collagenase injection in selected cases for functional improvement.

Anaesthetic techniques—general versus regional anaesthetic.

Post-surgical splintage and early rehabilitation with expert hand therapists. Supporting the patient with wound care and encouragement during the early healing phases.

7.3   Case 02

Pigmented and non-pigmented skin tumours in this same 69-year-old Caucasian woman living in a high sunlight region. The left scapular lesion shown in macro (Fig. 7.2a) and dermoscopic view (Fig. 7.2b) was confirmed as a superficial spreading malignant melanoma, Breslow thickness 0.6 mm with additional elements of in-situ melanoma. The pale nodule on the right mid helical rim (Fig. 7.2c) was an infiltrating basal cell carcinoma. The erythematous lesion lateral to the melanoma, just medial to her bra strap was also a BCC.

Questions could be asked testing the knowledge of diagnostic accuracy, excision margins, staging, sentinel node biopsy indications, specific dermatoscopic features, repair of defect to avoid tension and hypertrophic scarring, follow-up management and reconstruction of the helical rim to avoid deformity.

7.4   Cases 03, 04, 05

Three separate cases of congenital ear deformation. The first is a very prominent right ear due to relative unfolding of the antihelical fold. The second is cryptotia of the right ear where the upper pole is buried in the temporal scalp. The third is a double folding in the upper left helical rim with associated flattening. All three deformations were successfully treated with non-surgical ear moulding, which took from 4–12 weeks (Fig. 7.3).

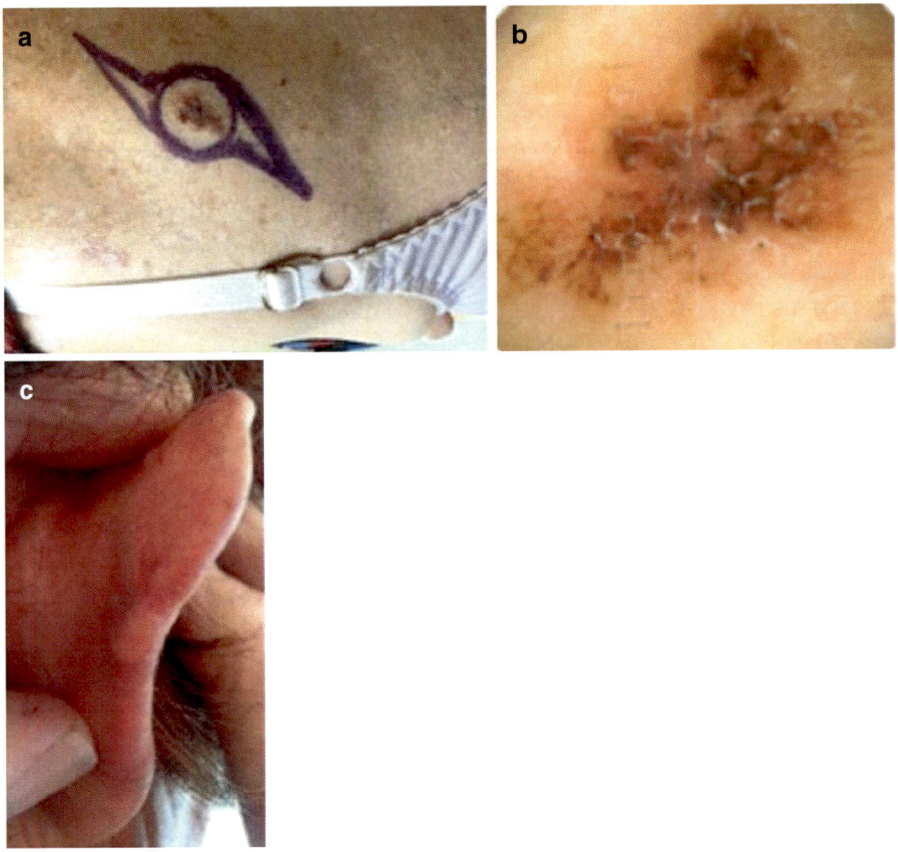

Fig. 7.2 (a) Shows gross images of melanoma left scapular region and (b), the dermatoscopic image of melanoma. (c) Shows an infiltrating non-pigmented BCC of her mid right helical rim

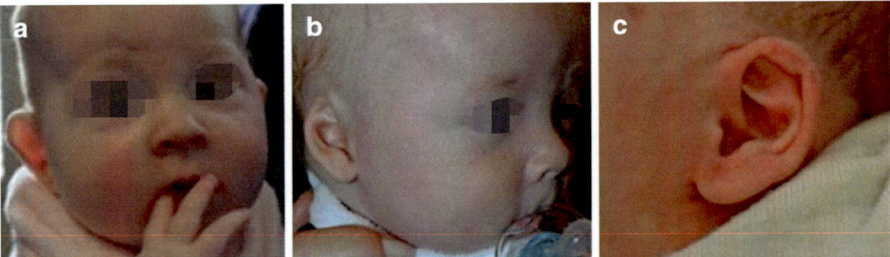

Fig. 7.3 (a) Shows a right prominent ear deformation in an infant, (b) is another type of deformation described as cryptotia (buried upper pole) and (c) is an example of kinked helical deformation

Ear moulding is very successful, particularly if applied early and ideally in the first 2 weeks of life. Twenty five percent of children who have normal looking ears at birth will develop prominent ears of varying severity. Up to 50% of babies may have some auricular deformation within 1 year of birth. Eighty six percent of ear deformations are noted by parents within the child's first 6 months of life.

Surgical otoplasty is not indicated until the child is at least 8 or 9 years of age and is motivated to have treatment. A general anaesthetic will be required for early surgical correction. Neonatal or infant ear moulding is cheap and easy, using lead-free soldering wire wrapped in Fixomull tape and fitted to the deformation with Steristrips or Micropore. Additional Fixomull is used to fix the splinted ear to the side of the head after limited hair removal. The splints are ideally changed every 2 weeks to check on skin hygiene. Commercial EarBuddies™ are also available.

7.5   Cases 06 and 07

Large keloid scars following ear piercing. The first case had previously undergone debulking and intralesional steroid injections 10 years previously. The second case had been treated by excision and full thickness postauricular skin graft 3 years previously. The modern treatment for such disfiguring and severe keloid scars is intralesional cryotherapy using a special delivery probe called the Cryoshape. This can be performed under local anaesthetic and is basically a frostbite induced necrosis of the keloid scar. The degree and extent of freezing requires training and experience, to be effective and not permanently damage soft tissues near the keloid (Fig. 7.4).

A discussion could ensue on the merits of the various techniques for management of keloids: intralesional steroid, excision and steroids, excision and radiation therapy, topical cryotherapy and finally the evidence for the efficacy of Cryoshape intralesional cryotherapy.

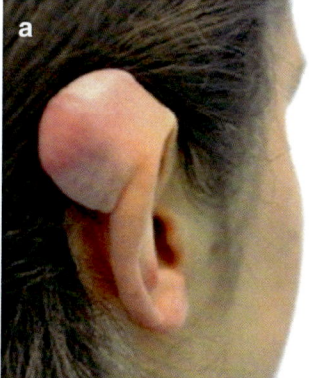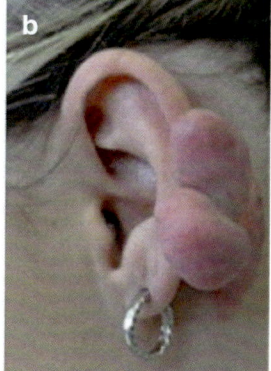

Fig. 7.4 (**a**) Is an example of a large recurrent keloid scar following ear-piercing. (**b**) Is a similar example of a keloid arising in an area of ear trauma

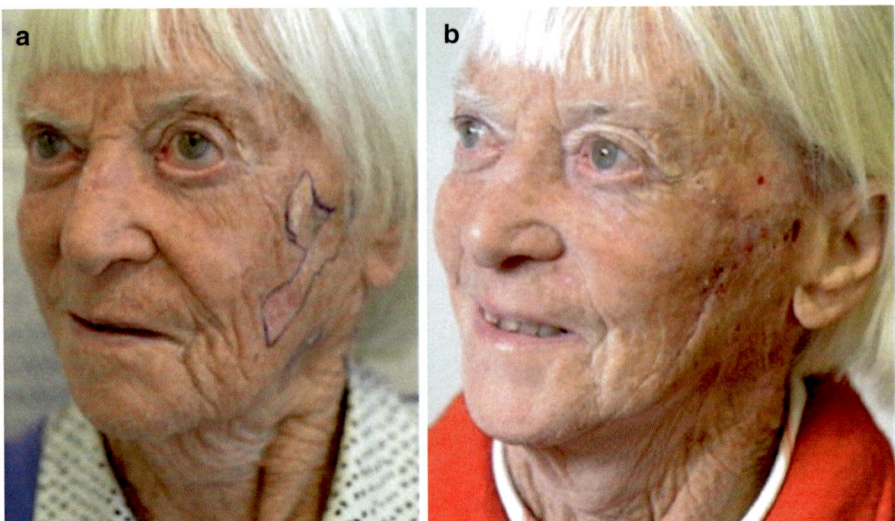

Fig. 7.5 (**a, b**) Show an 89-year-old lady before and after wide excision of multiple dysplastic SCC in-situ lesions involving her lateral cheeks, bilaterally. Repair with Flicklift advancement flaps

7.6   Case 08

An 89-year-old woman with lower eyelid laxity and retraction associated with severe photo-damage and a left lateral cheek complex of dysplastic actinic keratoses and multiple areas of squamous cell carcinoma in situ. *There is adequate lower face and neck skin laxity to achieve closure of the expected left cheek wound following surgical excision, but could this be combined with a lateral canthoplasty to reposition the lax lower eyelid?* (Fig. 7.5).

Discussions could develop with the differential diagnosis of the skin tumours (note also the actinic keratotic plaque on the dorsum nose) and also the various aetiologies of ectropion: senile, cicatricial and post-surgery. Inadvertent inferior tension on the lateral cheek skin could aggravate the lower lid ectropion. There also seems to be left facial asymmetry due either to a cerebrovascular incident or perhaps to previous skin tightening for a similar complex lesion on her contralateral cheek.

7.7   Case 09

A 55-year-old former rugby player with chronic subluxation of the proximal interphalangeal joint of his left non-dominant hand, resulting from recurrent dislocations including a compound dislocation. The PIPJ is permanently deviated 45 degrees in the ulnar direction and has almost 90 degrees of mal-alignment on

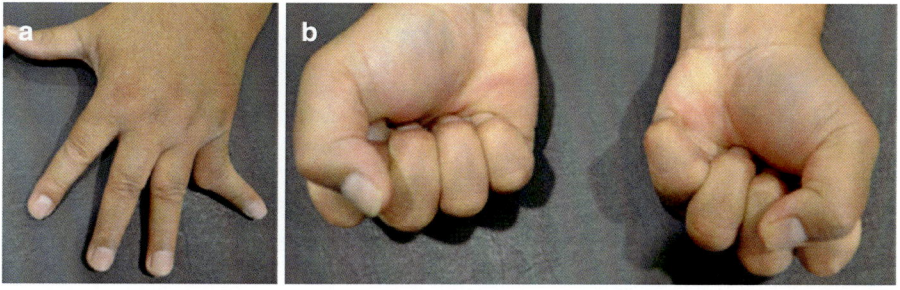

Fig. 7.6 (**a, b**) Show the chronically subluxing PIPJ of this 55-year-old former rugby player's left little finger. Compare his left little finger posture on making a fist, with his right hand

making a fist. The joint itself is stable and all the flexor and extensor tendons are functioning. Sensation and circulation are also normal (Fig. 7.6).

Is amputation a treatment option? What are the advantages and disadvantages?

A discussion on the best management plan would seem obvious. The current position of his little finger interferes with his ability to work without the risk of further injury. The options that could be considered are reconstructive arthroplasty versus functional arthrodesis, depending on bone stock and radiological status of the joint surfaces. Fusion in 40° of flexion after corrective osteotomies and fixation with a 3D miniplate and screws via a dorsal approach was the solution.

7.8   Case 10

This 59-year-old woman presents with an infiltrating BCC of her right nasal supratip. Biopsy excluded morphoeic features. Wide excision with a 3–5 mm margin is indicated respecting the nasal aesthetic subunits to achieve an aesthetic reconstruction according to the principle of CLEAR (refer Chap. 5). The predicted surgical defect overlaps the dorsum and right lateral sidewall subunits. Reconstructive options include a full thickness preauricular skin graft or a local nasoaxial advancement flap (based on left or right paranasal pedicle) with or without conservative reduction of the cartilaginous dorsum and large lateral alar crura. The introduction of aesthetic elements to the repair to achieve easier closure is a delicate issue, which requires a careful and respectful conversation. In this case the patient was delighted to combine her skin cancer removal with a conservative tip rhinoplasty. NB also shave excision of benign intradermal naevi (Fig. 7.7).

Skin cancers on the nose are common and this important landmark should be reconstructed with expertise to avoid disfigurement. A discussion could ensue on the merits of skin grafts versus local flaps, the role of Moh's surgery if any, and the problems seen with various bilobed and other poorly designed flaps, that disregard the aesthetic nasal subunits.

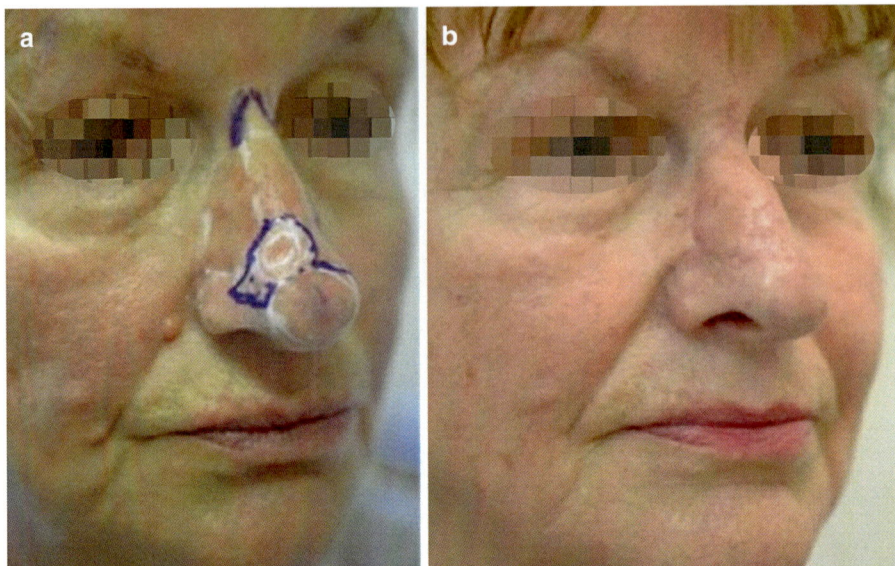

Fig. 7.7 (**a**) Shows a morphoeic infiltrating BCC of this 59-year-old woman's right nasal supratip / dorsum. (**b**) Shows the early result following wide excision and nasoaxial V-Y advancement local flap reconstruction

Scenarios: Surgical Pathology + Operative Surgery

8

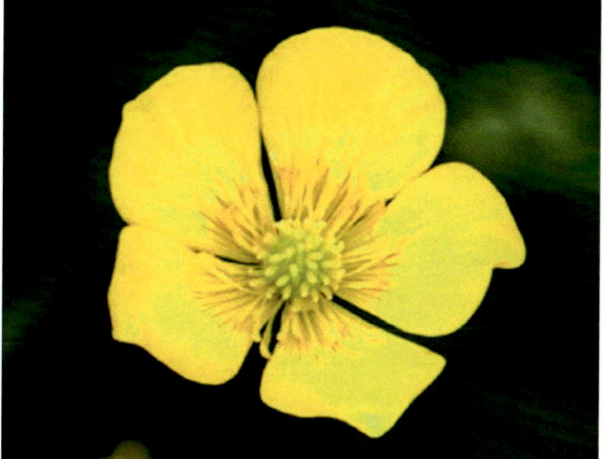

Ranunculus

Mediocrity is the jailor of freedom and the enemy of growth.
(John Fitzgerald Kennedy)

© Springer Nature Singapore Pte Ltd. 2018
M. F. Klaassen and E. Brown, *An Examiner's Guide to Professional Plastic Surgery Exams*, https://doi.org/10.1007/978-981-13-0689-1_8

8.1   Key Tips

1. Expect one trauma case and another complication case
2. Listen to the question—the emphasis may vary depending on the content of the rest of the Examination
3. If you cannot answer the question—best to say so. The examiner will move on. If it is a basic question, the examiner will re-direct the question in order to get the correct answer
4. A basic knowledge and interpretation of relevant histological slides is expected by the examiners

The scenarios of these oral examinations, known as 'Surgical Pathology & Operative Surgery' (SPOS), are two half-hour interactions, each with two examiners.

SPOS I consists of Scenarios, and SPOS II are clinical and pathology slides.

These two sessions tend to be complimentary to avoid any overlap of questions. The scenarios are mainly used for complications and trauma. They are perhaps the most difficult to prepare you for, because they are unpredictable and yet follow some standard clinical situations. It is in the scenarios that the candidate has the opportunity, to demonstrate all his or her skills of diagnosis, interpretation, clinical management and importantly, has the maturity to address unexpected clinical developments, complications and disasters.

Here are some mock clinical scenarios we have created to illustrate how you should communicate and perform to a successful standard:

8.2   Scenario 01 (Figs. 8.1, 8.2, 8.3, and 8.4)

Fig. 8.1 Shows the chronic venous ulcer on the lower shin of a 90-year-old lady. 3 months of intensive dressings have failed to achieve healing

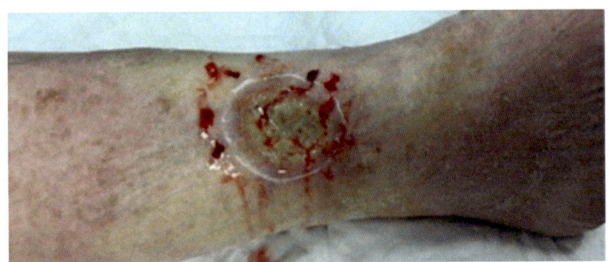

Examiners: This 90-year-old woman in a rest home with heart failure and mild dementia has a chronic painful ulcer for at least 3 months. Nurses are losing the treatment battle as the ulcer continues to grow in size and become more necrotic. What are your initial thoughts?

Necrotic ulcers, pressure sores and other wounds in very elderly patients are not uncommon problems, such as the chronic ulcer in this 90-year-old woman's left shin (Fig. 8.1). Sepsis from these wounds combined with multiple comorbidities can be potentially limb or life threatening. What are the real risks of proceeding with surgical debridement under local anaesthetic with minimal IV sedation versus the only other option of no treatment other than analgesia? What is the state of the peripheral circulation? Is diabetes a factor to consider? Is this a venous ulcer (most likely given the macroscopic appearance) or an arterial ulcer? Should malignancy be considered? How do you obtain informed consent, what do the family think?

The photographs show a white surgical marking pen line and blanching with bleeding needle points from local anaesthetic injection.

Which would be the safest local anaesthetic and what is the safe dose? Should an anaesthetist be present to give the IV sedation and what vital sign monitoring technology is available in the facility?

Fig. 8.2 Shows the ulcer following wide excision under local anaesthetic with a very light intravenous sedation

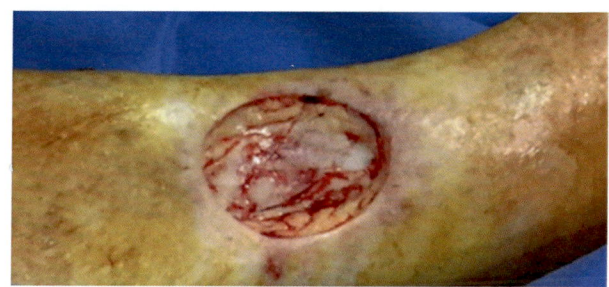

Examiners: The ulcer has been widely excised and debrided down to healthy periosteum over the lower anterior tibia. The defect measures 6 × 5 cm. She has tolerated this surgery well so far. What would you recommend next?

Half of the problem has been solved by removing the painful necrotic ulcer (Fig. 8.2).

Is there tissue missing?—YES.

Direct wound closure is clearly not possible. Local flap repair would necessitate a significant secondary defect which would require a skin graft.

A skin graft to the periosteum is a possibility but with a poor recipient bed. How can we buy some time with which to improve the blood supply?

Negative wound pressure devices come to mind, which will provide cover and prevent secondary infection. Are there any suitable allograft materials such as human amnion/chorion 'off-the-shelf' products, which may have a role combined with the negative wound pressure therapy? Would daily dressings with saline-soaked gauze, oral antibiotics and bed rest with leg elevation be a simpler solution?

Fig. 8.3 Shows the
application of an allograft
(Epifix derived from
placental tissue) plus
negative wound pressure
therapy device

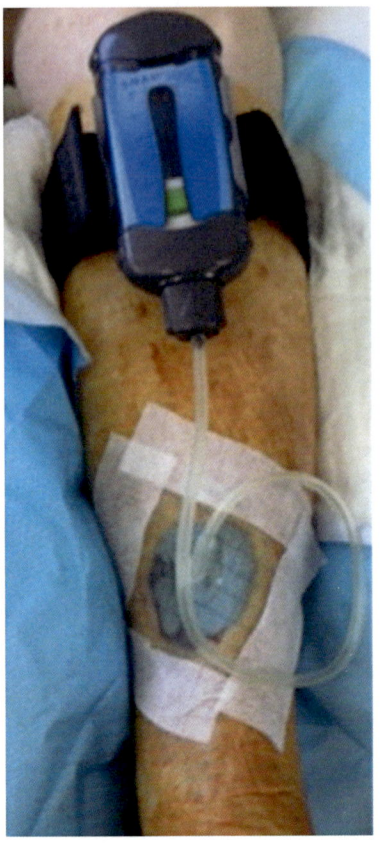

Discuss the mechanism by which negative wound therapy devices can help
manage chronic wounds? What added value would a product such as Epifix
(angiogenesis inducing homograft) bring to the management?

Negative pressure wound therapy induces healing by a number of synergistic
mechanisms including: increasing vascularity to the wound, removing waste and
toxic wound exudate products, forming a gentle closed occlusive dressing, inducing the early phases of wound healing and probably by a small biomechanical
expansion effect on the wound edges (Fig. 8.3). Many different forms of the
product are commercially available with various settings and device sizes, including the convenient minisystem shown above which can be strapped to the patient's
leg. This is the SNaP system which is based on a plunger negative pressure
action, which is simple and silent (no bleeps or annoying computer-driven
pumps). Special skills are required to fit and monitor the devices which nursing
staff are usually familiar with. The combination of tissue growth factors in the
homograft Epifix is growing in popularity but costs can be prohibitive as these
products are not cheap.

Fig. 8.4 Shows significant wound shrinkage and granulation formation at 10 weeks after surgical debridement

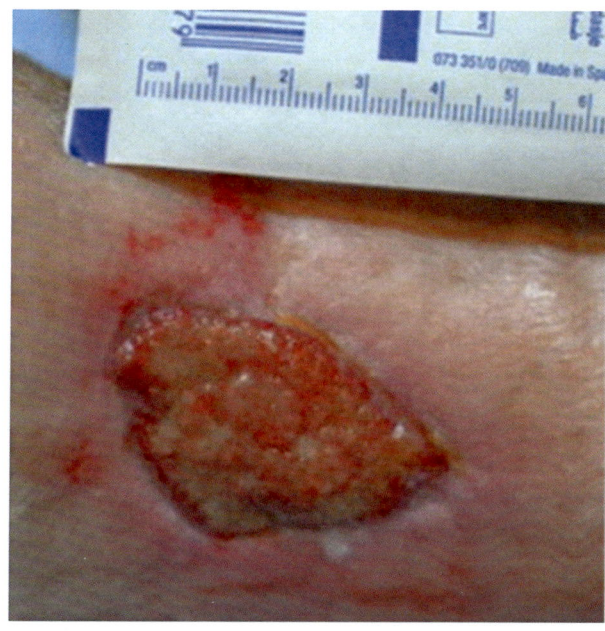

Examiners: This woman's ulcer is now 73 days post debridement. What are your comments? What else could you suggest?

There has been significant reduction in the ulcer size circumferentially in the last 10 weeks and healthy granulation tissue is seen filling the central defect (Fig. 8.4). The size of the wound is now approximately 4 × 3 cm compared to the initial 6 × 5 cm after surgical debridement, so this is definite, but slow progress. It is tempting to think about adding a thin split skin graft to the now vascularised wound bed but this would create a secondary defect and require another surgical procedure, however minor. You could suggest continuing with simple occlusive dressings with saline-soaked gauze, some topical antibiotic + low concentration steroid to discourage hypergranulation and/or the use of Silver Nitrate sticks for control of troublesome areas. Compression stockings over the dressing would also help with the venous hypertension in her leg and prevent further areas of ulceration. It would depend to a degree on the patient's comfort, the confidence of the nursing team to continue managing the wound (which they have done well to date) and ongoing conversations with the family at large.

8.3   Scenario 02 (Figs. 8.5, 8.6, 8.7, and 8.8)

Fig. 8.5 Shows a 39-year-old patient with functionally disabling bilateral severe breast hypertrophy. She wears an F cup brassiere

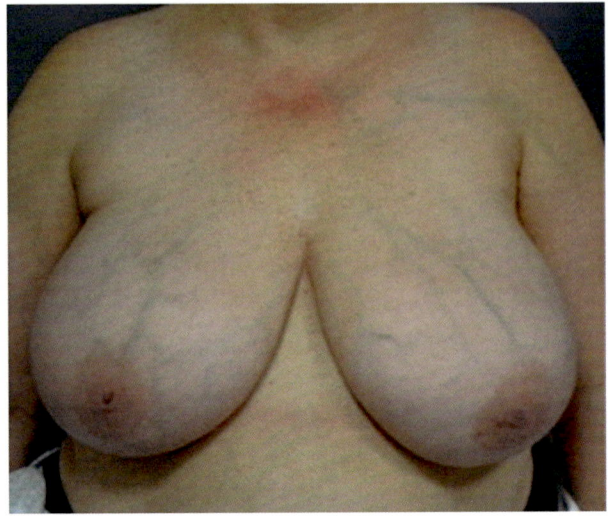

Examiners: This 39-year-old woman is concerned with her breast size and the functional problems it presents her. She runs her own business and is planning to marry her fiancé in 3 months.

Discuss your management plan?

What is the diagnosis?

What are her likely symptoms?

What method of surgery would you select for her?

Are there any concerns?

This is a case of severe breast hypertrophy in a young patient with relatively high BMI (Fig. 8.5). She would be suffering from the usual mechanical stresses of breast hypertrophy on her trunk, neck and back with pain and discomfort. Sleep disturbance and indigestion secondary to this degree of hypertrophy are symptomatic. This patient would certainly struggle to fit anything smaller than a G cup bra and other clothing issues may be a problem. She is probably self-conscious of this breast size as it may attract unwanted attention socially. Intertrigo problems, indentations from her bra straps and the engorged breast veins draining the nipple-areolar regions are other features which may concern her. A breast reduction technique combining liposuction and parenchymal resection is the best method for preserving the nipple-areolar complex on a reliable supra-medial dermoglandular pedicle. An aesthetic breast reduction could be planned so that she is healed and recovered in time for her eminent wedding. This is a large operation which could take 3–4 hours and the likely total resection weight would be >1.5 kg. Her high BMI adds to the surgical and anaesthetic risk factors.

Fig. 8.6 Reference markings and breast drawings for modified Lejour-style bilateral breast reduction

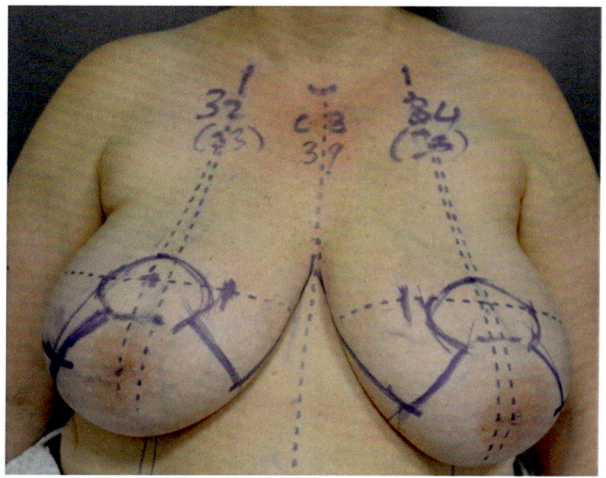

Examiners: Comment on the breast drawings? What are the important principles of planning a reduction mammoplasty?

The breast drawings highlight the asymmetry between each breast and also define the key reference planes—midline, breast meridian, inframammary fold level and the new proposed nipple-areola position along the corrected breast meridian (Fig. 8.6). The important principles are oncological, aesthetic and minimisation of wound healing complications. Both breasts should be examined and imaged for breast tumours. All resected tissue should be sent for histological examination. She is reaching a limit for potential pregnancy but outcome goals should include the need to preserve nipple function for lactation and erogenous sensation.

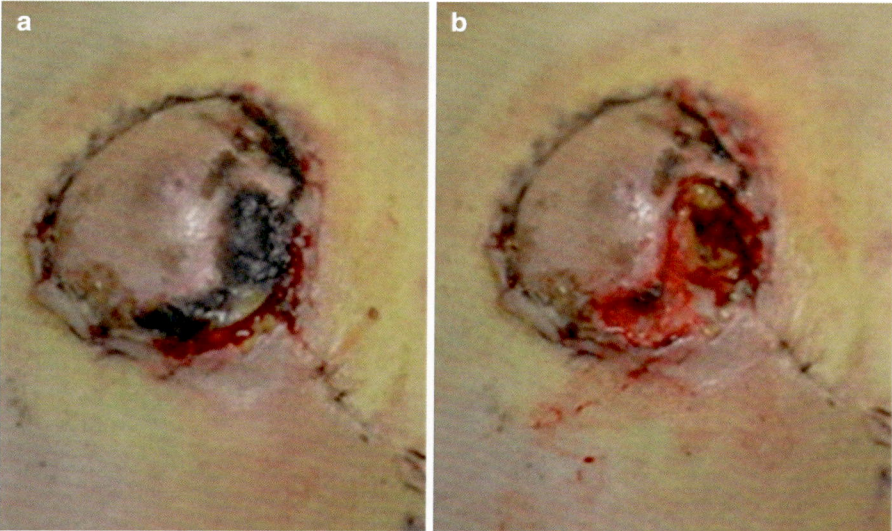

Fig. 8.7 (a) Shows early vascular insufficiency of the inferior areolar of the right NAC, and after scissor debridement in the clinic (b)

Examiners: This is the appearance of her right nipple-areolar complex 3 weeks after bilateral breast reduction. The left nipple-areola has healed without complication. Discuss the problem and how you would manage this?

This shows partial necrosis of the right infero-medial nipple areola complex probably due to venous insufficiency (Fig. 8.7). There may be associated partial fat necrosis. Debridement of the non-viable areola tissue has been performed in the second image. I would manage this conservatively with daily dressings, oral antibiotics and reassurance that this will heal spontaneously by secondary intention. I would maintain Micropore tape support for all her other healed breast scars and also encourage her to wear a surgical bra for support night and day for another month.

Fig. 8.8 Shows both breasts healed at 2 months post surgery

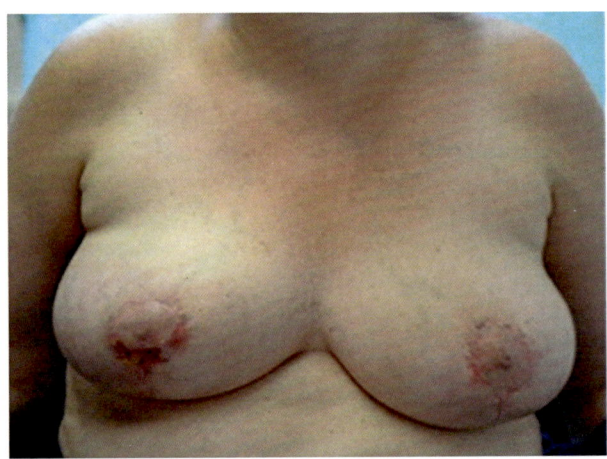

Examiners: This is the patient's appearance two months post bilateral breast reduction with a modified Lejour vertical mammoplasty. Discuss the early result and make some comments about the aftercare of patients having breast reduction surgery?

The breasts have now healed but the scars are still somewhat hypertrophic (Fig. 8.8). Some asymmetry remains with the left breast still being larger than the right. The absence of medial breast scars, characteristic of the Lejour vertical mammoplasty is a bonus. The early result at 2 months shows some bottoming out, but her breasts are still at least a C–D cup bra size in balance with her general body habitus.

8.4   **Scenario 03** (Figs. 8.9, 8.10, 8.11, and 8.12)

Fig. 8.9 Shows the notch deformity resulting from failed local nasolabial flap repair of right nostril defect, post BCC excision

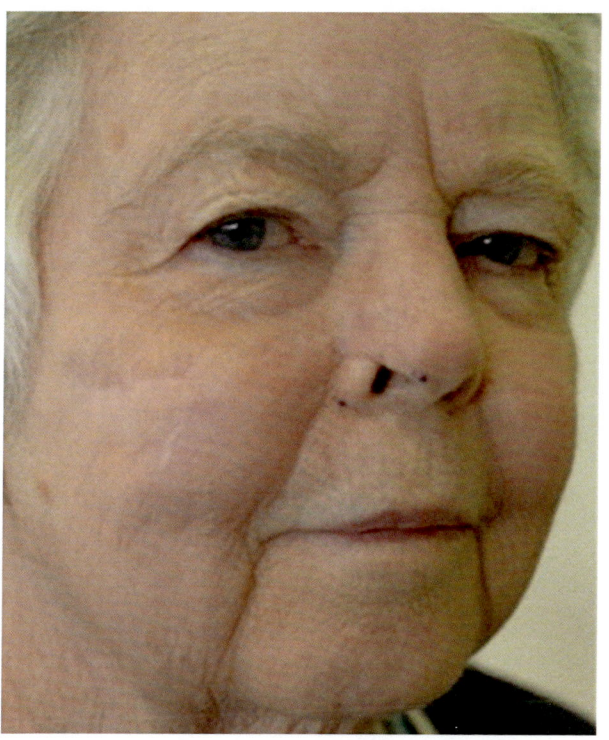

Examiners: This 74-year-old woman presents to you with a notch deformity of her right alar region. Six months previously her GP had excised a BCC close to the right alar rim and attempted repair with a superiorly-based nasolabial flap. There were questions from the pathologist about adequacy of excision margins so a redo excision was performed and subsequently the distal end of the local flap necrosed. She also has a high mid cheek scar, which appears to cross the relaxed skin tensions lines and this again was a previous local flap repair after BCC excision.

What would you recommend to improve her situation?

The first choice treatment of moderate sized nasal alar defects is an extended composite graft taken from a helical rim (Fig. 8.9). The tongue of skin in continuity with the harvested graft is de-epithelialised and buried under the side-wall of the nose to enhance the vascularisation of the graft.

A W-plasty of her anti-RSTL cheek scar could also be considered.

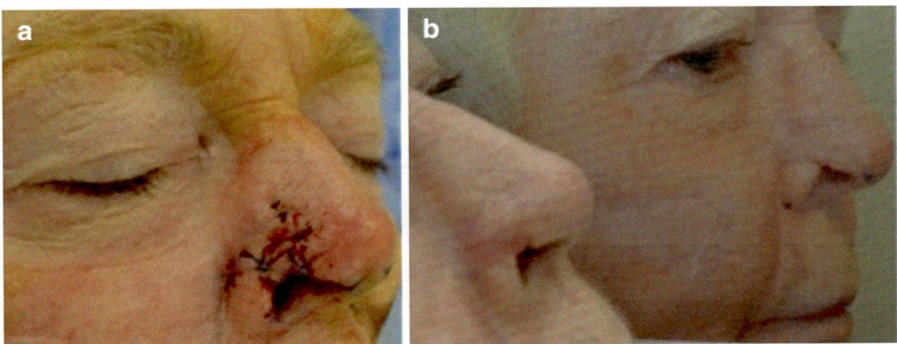

Fig. 8.10 (**a**) Shows attempted salvage of the poor reconstruction with an auricular composite flap. (**b**) shows the less than 'perfect' result. A lifeboat is needed

Examiners: A composite auricular graft has been attempted to correct the right alar notch and the result at 6 months is shown. Comment and advise?

The selected composite graft was probably inadequate in size and there has been partial failure of the graft (Fig. 8.10). Although an improvement, the final result at 6 months is still less than perfect.

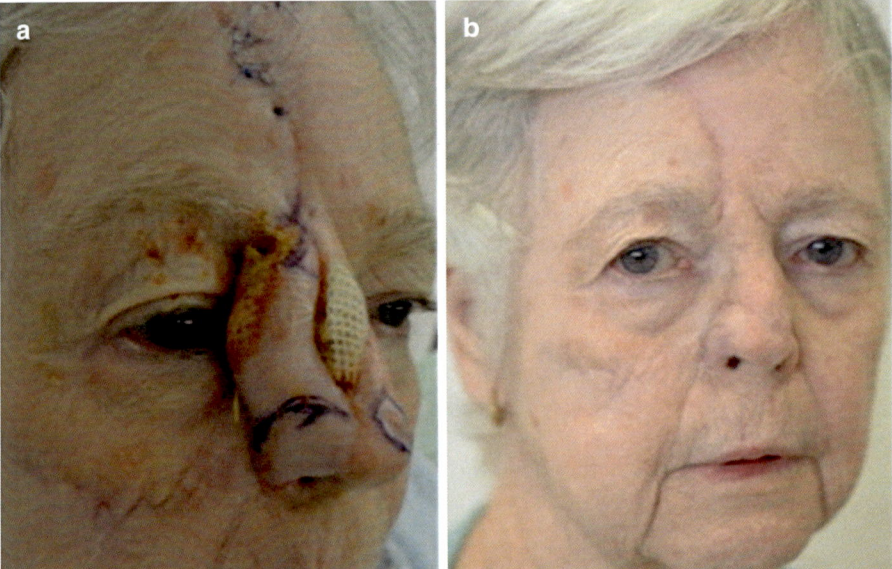

Fig. 8.11 (**a**) Demonstrates the right paramedian forehead flap used to salvage the right nostril reconstruction. Auricular cartilage graft was placed beneath the flap for nostril support. (**b**) shows early result after division and inset

Examiners: A year later after salvage with a staged paramedian forehead flap the patient is shown now aged 76 years.

Discuss the principles of staged nose reconstruction in this specific case?

Would you offer her any further revisions?

There was both tissue missing and tissue displaced in the notched right alar defect following BCC excision and only partial success of the composite graft (Fig. 8.11). Nasal reconstruction requires lining, support and cover. The internal mucosal lining of her right alar defect could be constructed with either a septal lining flap or a turnover flap from the distal end of the paramedian forehead flap. This latter flap is the ideal tissue for cover, planned in reverse and supported by a contoured conchal cartilage graft from her right ear. This would be a two-stage procedure performed under general anaesthesia with an overnight hospital stay. The second stage, to divide and inset the flap would be planned for at least 2 weeks after the first stage. A third stage may be necessary after at least 3 months to refine the aesthetic reconstruction and achieve near perfection.

This involved thinning of the forehead flap alar reconstruction and the re-creation of a neo alar crease (Fig. 8.12). A new actinic lesion in the right orbital region below the eyebrow was excised at this time (Fig. 8.12).

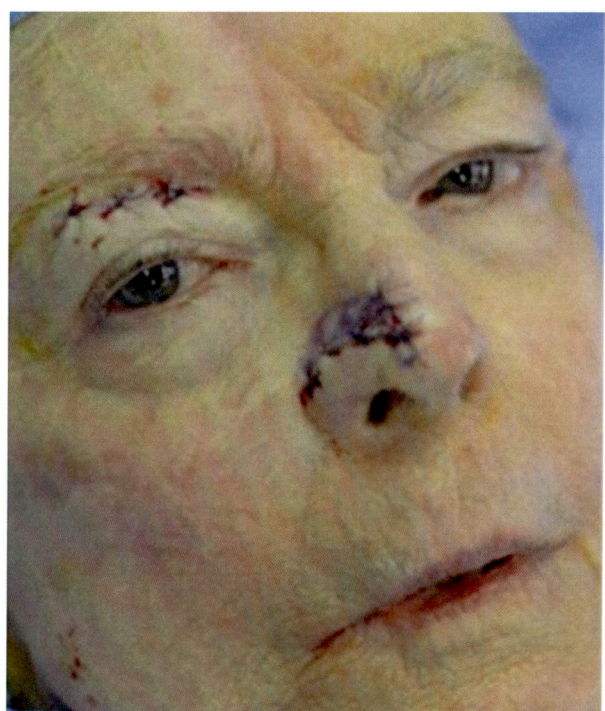

Fig. 8.12 Shows the immediate result after the third stage to recreate the right alar crease

8.5   Scenario 04 (Figs. 8.13, 8.14, 8.15, and 8.16)

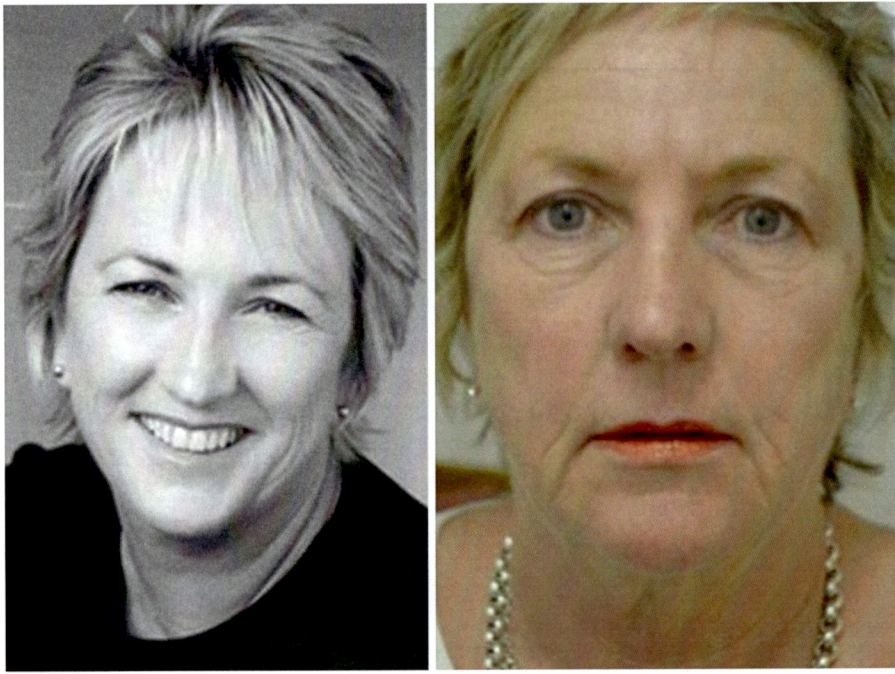

Fig. 8.13 Shows a woman aged 49 years and ten years later when she is requesting facial rejuvenation surgery aged 59 years

Examiners: This 59-year-old woman is referred to you for facial rejuvenation. She is healthy but 5 years before after a bilateral breast reduction she developed an acute breast haematoma, which required emergency drainage and evacuation. She wants to look fresher and more youthful like she used to ten years before (Fig. 8.4a).
     Discuss your management?
She looks like a good candidate for a facelift to correct her tired look and classic stigmata including: brow ptosis, dermatochalasia of her upper eyelids, tear trough deformity of the lower eyelid/mid cheek junctions, flattening and loss of convexity in her malar regions, associated atrophy of the soft tissue in her periorbital and temporal regions, early jowls and marionette lines, loose neck and loss of definition of her jawline and sternomastoid contour (Fig. 8.13). I would be concerned about the prior history of post-surgical bleeding and look into this critically as part of her pre-operative assessment. Does she have a coagulation disorder or is she taking anticoagulants? I would ask her what her motivations and expectations were. I would document a surgical plan with annotation of photographs and produce a careful informed clinical and financial consent. I would encourage her to reflect on all this in a 'cooling down' period of at least 4–6 weeks. I would plan to see her again at no further charge to discuss her concerns, questions and decisions whenever this suited her. I would ask if I could communicate also with her family doctor/GP who should know her well. I would show her previous facelift cases on PowerPoint, with a variety of methods and balance this with good, bad and indifferent results achieved by my hands, including actual complications.

Fig. 8.14 Shows the same patient one week after a conservative facelift with bilateral infected preauricular haematomata

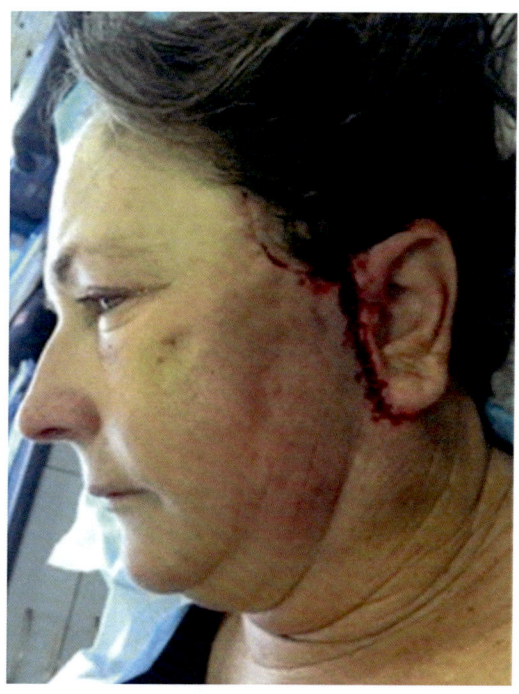

Examiners: The facelift surgery including upper lid blepharoplasty is uneventful and she is discharged home the following day. She returns at 7 days post surgery complaining of bilateral wound discharge, pain and fever. She is unwell. This is the appearance of her left hemiface at 7 days. What is your impression?

What will you do next?

What will you tell the patient?

The diagnosis is bilateral infected late haematomata (Fig. 8.14). It requires urgent release and evacuation either in my clinic treatment room under local anaesthetic (if possible) or else a return to the operating theatre and general anaesthetic. I would wash out the wounds, take swabs and pack the wounds with saline + dilute Betadine soaked wet gauze swabs. I would change these daily for the next week at least. I would tell her that this is a serious complication and apologise for the inconvenience, but reassure her that I am available 24/7 and I will do everything in my skill set to salvage the situation and get her healed. I would warn her that there would be a period of regular dressings and perhaps 3–6 months down the track revision of scars. I would stress that she has paid for her surgery already and there would be no further charges from me, but hospital charges may be a possibility. I would document and photograph her progress weekly. I would inform her GP and organise specialist nurses of my practice to help with the aftercare. She would have my email, personal phone number and my secretaries personal number so that she could call us anytime. I would tell her that we are going to become the best of friends because we'll be seeing a lot of each other over the next few weeks. I would put aside extra clinic time for conversations and explanatory reassuring discussions with her and her family.

Don't go on vacation and leave this problem for another colleague to manage. Take full responsibility and don't make excuses for the complication.

Fig. 8.15 Shows the
clinical situation post
haematoma evacuation,
washout with betadine/
saline, daily dressings and
oral antibiotics four weeks
post her initial facelift
surgery

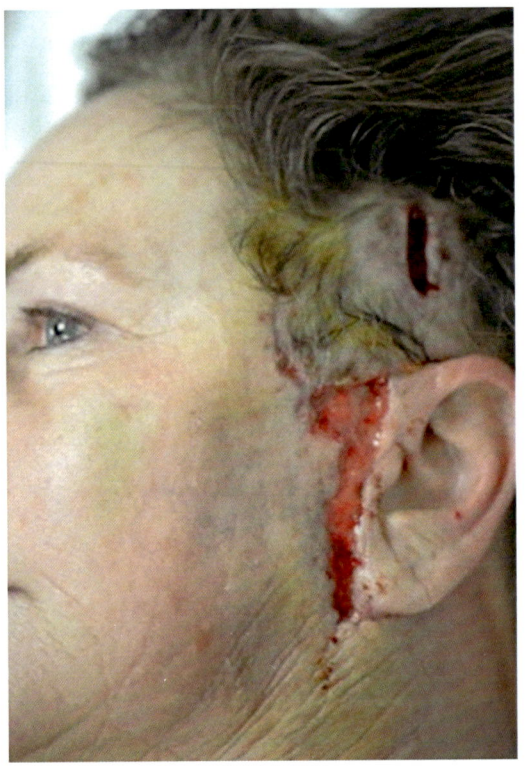

Examiners: This is the appearance of her left hemiface at 4 weeks post bilateral facelift surgery. The right hemiface has similar granulating open wounds of the preauricular and temporal regions.

What would be your management now?

What would you tell the patient?

What is the likely outcome?

She made excellent progress in the context of a major complication (Fig. 8.15). Infection has resolved and dehisced preauricular wounds are now granulating. Hypergranulation may be a problem soon so I would be ready to add silver nitrate topically or Soframycin (antibiotic/steroid mix). I would remove any obvious permanent sutures in the depths of the wounds if they were visible. I would tell the patient that she is now a star healer and progress is as good as I could have expected. I would have conversations with her trying to ascertain if anxiety and or depression as a result of the castastrophe is an issue. I would remain positive and supportive. Serial photographs if she can bare to look at them would be documenting the recovery. I would suggest to her that sometime, we may need to investigate her haematological status more formally with more advanced clotting tests and perhaps even a clinical haematological opinion. These investigations are indicated in view of her previous history of post-surgery haematoma (breast reduction). I would continue to see her weekly or as often as she required. I would keep in touch with any attending nurses and be briefed by them. Regular follow-up reports in writing to the patient and her GP.

Fig. 8.16 Same patient healed an happy at 3 months post facelift surgery

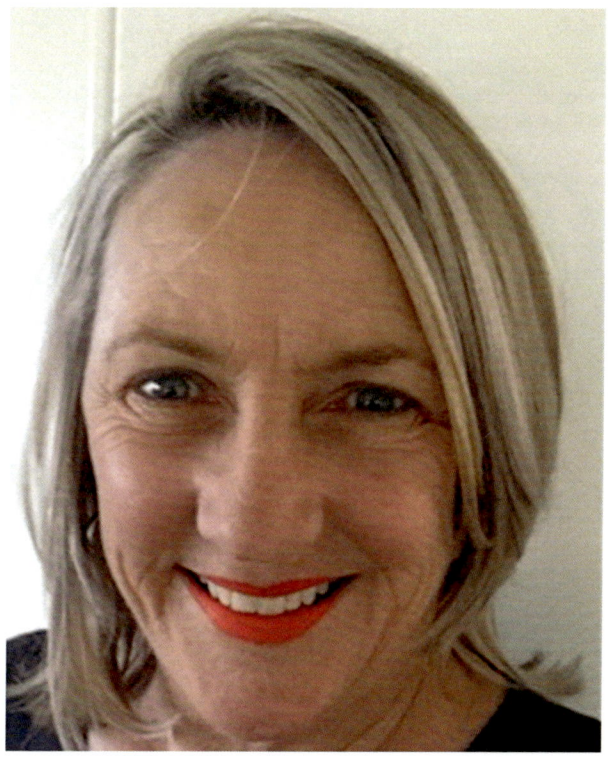

Examiners: Same patient at 12 months post bilateral facelift with complications. What would you advise now and going forward over the next 6 – 12 months?

She is healed and looking good! (Fig. 8.16) There is some residual neck laxity and there may be a need for some maintenance procedures to the neck including the modified Fogli total neck lift of Dr. Darryll Hodgkinson in 6 months to a year, depending on her wishes. I would see her again in 2 months, then 3 months and again a year following her initial surgery. I would refer her for formal haematological assessment.

8.6   Scenario 05 (Figs. 8.17 and 8.18)

Fig. 8.17 Shows a 56-year-old woman marked up pre-surgery for a necklift

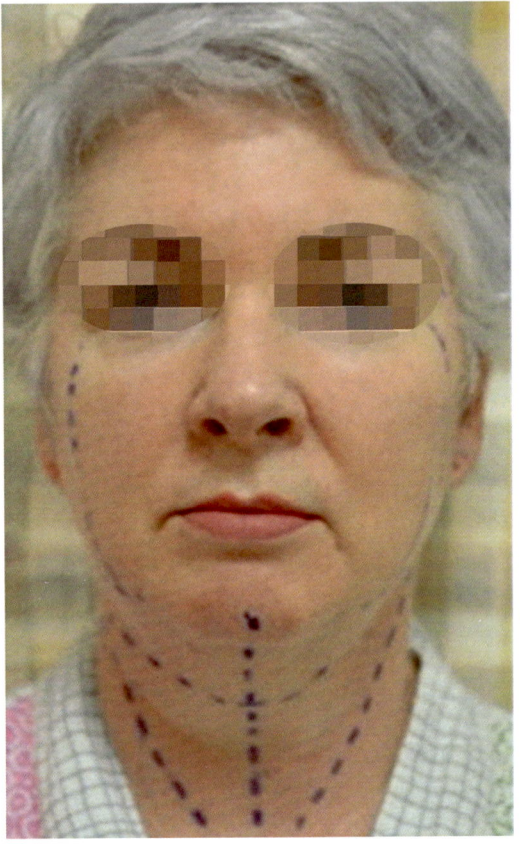

Examiners: This 56-year-old woman is marked up for a necklift only. She is concerned about her heavy neck and submental laxity. She is not concerned about her mid and upper face.

Discuss you plan for a cosmetic necklift?

This woman has attractive full contours of her upper face and attention should focus on her lower face and neck (Fig. 8.17). The dotted reference lines indicate the vertical midline, the major facial pilaster transitioning from the frontal plane to the lateral facial planes and also in the neck the level of the hyoid bone and the anterior surface landmark of sternocleidomastoid muscle. I would use a fine cannula suction-assisted liposuction technique to debulk the fat in her neck, then I would through a limited preauricular and temporal incision expose enough of SMAS and platysma to execute a SMAS/Platysma plication anchored to her deep temporal fascia with strong non-absorbable 2/0 sutures. I would manage her in a soft cervical collar for 2 weeks to restrict neck movement and I would probably use neck drains that could be removed at 24–48 h.

Fig. 8.18 Same patient one month post neck liposuction and conservative necklift, with lower lip asymmetry

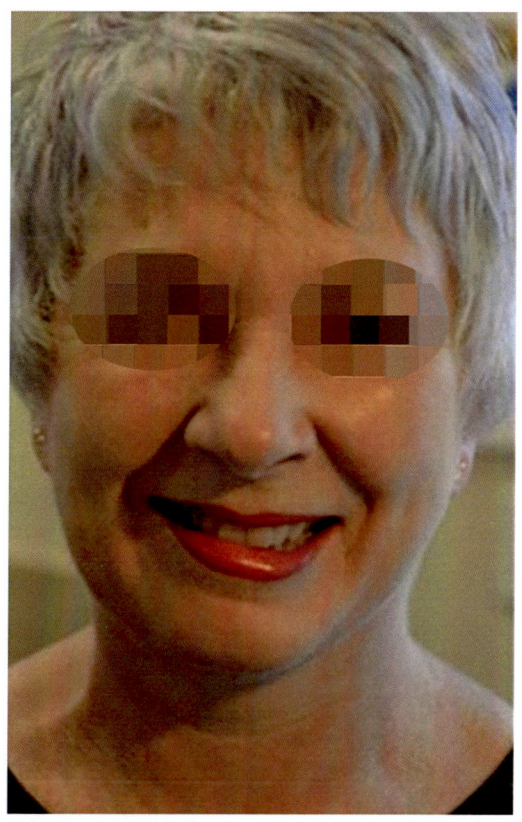

Examiners: This is the same patient a month post necklift surgery. The procedure involved initial liposuction followed by a SMAS-Plastyma plication with purse-string sutures anchored to her deep temporal fascia.

She is aware of asymmetry when she smiles.

What is the diagnosis?

What would you tell the patient?

How would you manage this?

The diagnosis is damage to the right marginal mandibular branch of the seventh cranial nerve with inability to depress her right lower lip (Fig. 8.18). Depressor labii inferioris muscle is the main culprit here, but depressor anguli oris is also at risk. This is either due to iatrogenic injury perioperatively, due to liposuction cannula trauma, traction injury or catching branches of the nerve with the plication sutures. Most likely it is a neuropraxic injury and will spontaneously resolve over the next 3 months. If there was no recovery by 6 months I would investigate with nerve conduction studies and EMG before planning to perform an anterior belly of digastric transfer. This facial muscle is innervated by the fifth cranial nerve. I would be completely open to the patient about what has happened, what this means and what I can do to improve the problem. Reassurance and close follow-up are the key strategies for management. The neuropraxic marginal mandibular branch nerve injury completely recovered by 3 months.

8.7   Scenario 06 (Figs. 8.19, 8.20, and 8.21)

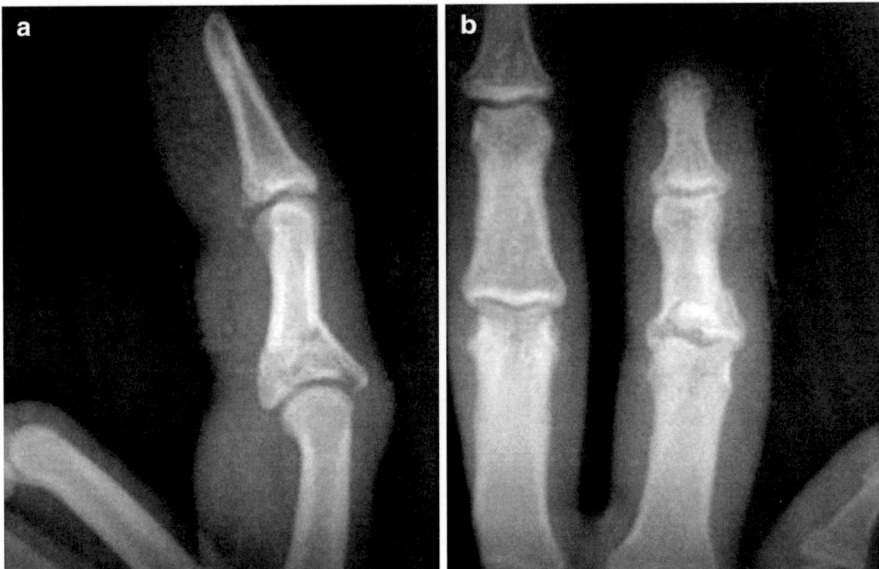

Fig. 8.19 Plain X-Ray images of the left dominant index finger of a 23-year-old cricket who sustained a direct blow and axial compression forces, from a fast moving cricket ball, earlier in the day

Fig. 8.20 Shows the CT scan radiological appearance from a lateral view

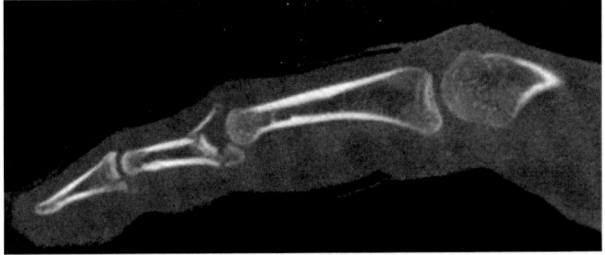

Examiners: These are the initial plain X-Rays of a 23-year-old male cricket player who has been struck on the tip of his dominant left index finger, by the hard cricket ball, whilst trying to make a caught-and-bowled catch, close to the batsman.

Diagnosis?

Investigations?

Management?

This is a comminuted intra-articular pilon fracture of the base of his middle phalanx and PIPJ from an axial compression force to his dominant left index finger. The DIPJ also has signs of injury, probably an avulsion fracture and dislocation, which has already been reduced. This is a severe injury and potentially a cricket career-ending injury. Expert management in a multidisciplinary of specialist hand unit is the ideal. A CT scan demonstrates the pathology.

Fig. 8.21 Shows the CT
radiological view from the
AP view

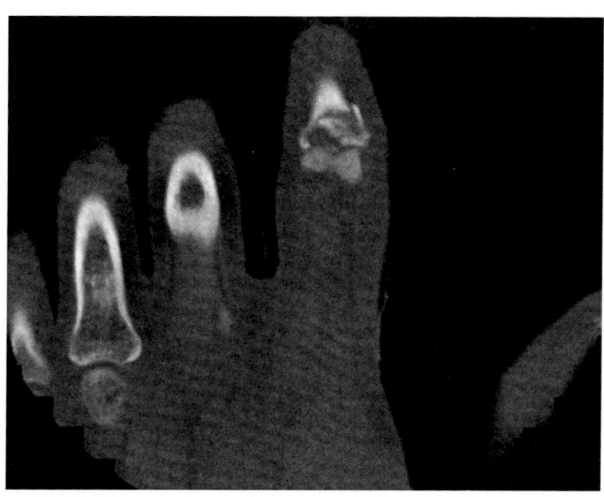

Selected CT scans for detail of the injury.
Discuss your management plans including post-operative rehabilitation?
What is the prognosis for him returning to first class cricket?

Surgical options include: ORIF with miniplates and screws, formal arthrodesis
of the PIPJ in functional flexion or reconstruction using a distraction device (Suzuki
frame) with bone grafting of the base of the middle phalanx. This latter approach
preserves remaining articular cartilage fragments and once bone union is achieved
an intensive programme of hand therapy and rehabilitation begins. There is perhaps a 50:50 chance of returning to top level cricket for this patient. Patient motivation and compliance probably account for 70% of the final outcome.

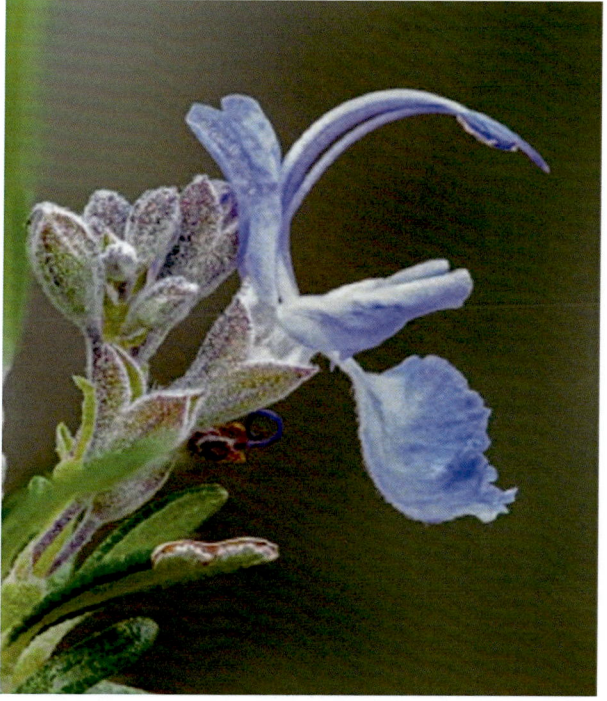

Rosemary

What we know is not much. What we don't know is enormous.

(Pierre-Simon Laplace)

© Springer Nature Singapore Pte Ltd. 2018
M. F. Klaassen and E. Brown, *An Examiner's Guide to Professional Plastic Surgery Exams*, https://doi.org/10.1007/978-981-13-0689-1_9

9.1   Key Tips

1. Questions tend to be on functional and applied anatomy
2. Common embryological questions would be on the mandible and branchial clefts
3. Knowledge of flap anatomy of the whole body is essential
4. Orientate the anatomical specimen before identifying the specific structure
5. Practice anatomy questioning, as you would for the long and short clinical cases

Applied anatomy is the foundation of surgery. For the final fellowship exams in plastic surgery it is the comprehensive working knowledge of gross and micro-anatomy from the head-to-foot, and everything in between. Surface and functional anatomy, aesthetic landmarks, important vital structures, dissection planes, surgical approaches and the specific anatomy of local, loco-regional, pedicled and free flaps are the syllabus. Some details of osteology, embryological anatomy and anatomical anomalies are also considered.

9.2   Surface and Functional Anatomy

1. The superficial temporal, occipital and supratrochlear branches of the carotid vascular system.
2. The location of the supraorbital, infraorbital and mental sensory nerves.
3. The location and approach to the main branch of the facial nerve.
4. The terminal branches of the facial artery.
5. The location and preservation of the greater auricular nerve.
6. The radial and ulnar vascular pedicles.
7. The posterior radial collateral pedicle.
8. The origin of the thoraco-acromial axis and its pectoral branches.
9. The circumflex scapular and thoracodorsal pedicles.
10. The deep inferior epigastric pedicle.
11. The superficial and deep circumflex iliac pedicles.
12. The descending branch of the lateral circumflex femoral pedicle.
13. The peroneal nerve and peroneal pedicle.
14. The sural artery and nerve.
15. The lateral tarsal branch of dorsalis pedis.
16. The medial plantar pedicle [1].

9.3   Aesthetic Landmarks

1. The facial dimensions and congruent contours
2. The brow and hairline symmetry
3. The lower eyelid/cheek junction contours

4. The malar prominence
5. The medial cheeks—nasolabial folds and jowls
6. The lateral cheeks and the Obaji cheek profile
7. The cupid's bow/philtral column relationships
8. The nasal aesthetic subunits and contours
9. The chin point and submental regions/cervicomental angle
10. The neck length and contour including the suprasternal notch and sternomastoid definition

9.4   Osteology

1. The facial bones
2. The mandible
3. The skull base
4. The first rib
5. The scapula
6. The radius
7. The ulnar
8. The bones of the hand and wrist
9. The ilium
10. The fibula

9.5   Surgical Approaches

1. To the temporomandibular joint
2. To the infratemporal fossa
3. To the orbit
4. To the nasal cavity
5. To the maxilla
6. To the mandible
7. To the various zones of the neck
8. Tracheostomy (emergency and elective)
9. To the thoracic duct
10. To the brachial plexus
11. To the ulnar, radial and median nerves
12. Hand anatomy
13. Rib cartilage harvest
14. Internal mammary pedicle
15. To delay a TRAM flap
16. Origin and branches of the DIEP flap
17. Sciatic nerve
18. Fasciotomy for limb compartment syndrome

9.6   Local and Regional Flaps (Pedicled and Free)

1. Scalp rotation, transposition and keystone local flaps
2. Forehead flaps
3. Cervicofacial flaps
4. Nasolabial and FAMM flaps
5. Fan and Karapandzic flaps + Bernard flaps
6. Submental flaps
7. Trapezius flaps
8. Delto-pectoral flaps
9. Pectoralis major and minor flaps
10. Latissimus dorsi flaps (antegrade and reverse)
11. Lateral arm flap
12. Forearm flaps (radial, ulnar and posterior interosseous)
13. Dorsal metacarpal flap
14. Rectus abdominis (pedicled, free and perforator flaps)—TRAM, VRAM, ORAM, DIEP
15. The groin flap
16. DCIA flap
17. TFL flap
18. Gluteus maximus flap
19. Anterolateral thigh flap
20. Saphenous flap
21. Gastrocnemius flaps (medial and lateral)
22. Soleus flap
23. Fibula flap
24. Reverse sural artery flap
25. Dorsalis pedis flap
26. Extensor digitorum brevis flap
27. Great toe flaps (wrap around composite flap of Morrison)
28. Medial plantar fasciocutaneous flap of Morrison

9.7   Knowledge of Dermatomes

A dermatome is defined as an area of skin supplied by nerves from a single spinal root.

Behan et al. have shown that island fasciocutaneous flaps can be safely and predictably raised based on a knowledge of the dermatomal anatomy. Vessels travel with nerves (motor and sensory) and therefore the dermatomes can be used as an aide memoire or road map for localisation of the many named and unnamed, random or axial, perforators. This provides improved vascularity and healing with reduced risk of complications.

The angiotome concept evolved from the understanding that the trilaminate composition of skin, fat and fascia supplied by fasciocutaneous, musculocutaneous or septocutaneous vessels can be designed as reconstructive flaps based on vascular and neural anatomy. The term ANGIOTOME refers to a vascularised segment with an axial input, which can be extended in size by its communications with adjacent vessels. Behan first started applying this principle to reconstructive limb challenges in the 1970s and 1980s.

Taylor et al. developed the concept of angiosome in-vitro based on an extensive number of cadaver injection studies. The ANGIOSOME refers to the 3D block of tissue supplied by a source vessel directly or indirectly. The difference between angiotome and angiosome concepts is subtle, but the critical principle is that flaps based on the angiotomal theory do not require dermal connections. They are islanded on their fasciocutaneous perforators and there is a predictable and observable hyperaemic phase. This may be due to a denervation, sympathectomy or metabolic effects.

The role of dermatomes is again noted in the description of various named flaps:
Groin flap L1 dermatome.
Radial forearm flap C6, C7.
Lateral arm flap C6, C7, C8.
Medial instep flap L 5.

9.8 Embryological Development

The candidates should have a working knowledge of the embryological anomalies for the anatomical regions listed. The relevance of this to clinical reconstructive challenges is a key concept for exam preparation and potential discussion with te examiners.
Face.
Limbs.
Hand.
Genitalia.

9.9 Anatomy of Common Flaps

9.9.1 Temporalis Flap [2]

This flap was originally described by Golovine in 1898. The origin of the temporalis muscle is from the temporal fossa and the deep surface of the temporal fascia and its converging fibres end in a tendon inserted in to the coronoid process of the mandible. Its blood supply is from two deep temporal arteries and venae comitantes deep to the muscle. The nerve supply is from the deep temporal branches of the mandibular nerve. The flap is raised via a hemicoronal incision and can be designed as muscle only, muscle + galea and muscle + bone. Clinical uses include: orbit, midface, skull base, palate and pharynx and facial reanimation for facial palsy. The temporalis muscle can be used for filling an exenterated orbit and the pedicled temporalis fascia for covering the cartilage construct of an ear reconstruction.

The temporal fascia can also be used as a new ligament for the TMJ following dislocations.

9.9.2 Forehead Flap [3]

The original application of this flap was by Susruta in 600 BC for nasal reconstruction. The First World War saw widespread use of this flap by Plastic surgery pioneers Gillies and Pickerill, for nasal and facial reconstruction of severe facial injuries. Forehead flaps can be of many designs based on the rich vascular network of superficial temporal vessels laterally and supratrochlear and supraorbital vessels medially. Variations include: paramedian, total forehead, prefabricated and tissue expanded forms of the forehead flap. Some frontalis muscle fibres should be left where the pedicles emerge from the skull. Clinical uses include: nose reconstruction, eyelid reconstruction and potentially intra oral reconstruction.

9.9.3 Facial Artery Flaps [4]

Flaps based on branches of the facial artery have been described since 1881. The majority of these apply to the facial skin, but a musculo-mucosal flap has also been described by Pribaz in 1992, the FAMM flap (Facial Artery Musculo-Mucosal flap). The tortuous facial artery and accompanying venae comitantes follow the nasolabial fold deep to the mimetic muscles and superficial to the buccinator masticatory muscle. The superior labial branch arises at the corner of the mouth and the terminal branch is the angular artery towards the medial canthal region. Skin nasolabial flaps for lower nose and columellar reconstruction, superiorly or inferiorly based, are common repairs in facial surgery and can be in single or two stages.

The musculo-mucosal flap should be designed anterior to Stenson's duct, extending from retromolar trigone to the labial sulcus at the level of the nasal alar margin. It is useful in intra-oral reconstruction of the hard palate, floor of mouth, lip and ventral tongue for small defects.

9.9.4 Cervicofacial Flaps [5]

Esser first described this rotation flap in the German literature, in 1918. Frame and Levick described their Anterior Flicklift flap in 2012 for facial rejuvenation and it has recently (2017) been described for reconstructive problems. Many variations of cervicofacial flaps are possible based on the extensive random pattern blood supply, including the perialar crescentic advancement flaps of Webster (1955). The facelift plane does not need to include SMAS or platysma as demonstrated by Pennington and Poole. Small or large cutaneous defects of the hemiface, lower eyelid/cheek junction, malar and preauricular regions can be repaired with these flaps.

9.9.5 Supraclavicular Flap [6]

Lamberty described this axial-patterned fasciocutaneous flap in 1979. The supraclavicular artery is a branch of the transverse cervical artery in the neck at the midclavicular level. The latter artery arises from the thyrocervical trunk and supplies trapezius muscle. The supraclavicular artery runs laterally towards the acromioclavicular joint where it can anastomose with branches of the posterior circumflex humeral vessels. The flap can be islanded and is very useful in head and neck reconstruction including neck scar contractures.

9.9.6 Trapezius Flap [7]

McCraw et al. described this flap in 1979 for head and neck reconstruction. The trapezius muscle myocutaneous flap is a broad triangular muscle arising from the cervicothoracic vertebrae and inserting into the spine of the scapula. The transverse cervical artery is the blood supply (with ascending and descending branches), and the spinal accessory nerve (XI) the motor nerve. It can be used as either a muscle flap or a musculocutaneous flap for large defects of the posterior neck and occipital area. The large donor site is best closed with a keystone perforator island local flap.

9.9.7 Deltopectoral Flap [8]

Bakamijian described this pectoral skin flap for pharyngoesophageal reconstruction in 1965. It is an axial-patterned fasciocutaneous flap based on the second and third intercostal branches of the internal mammary artery, arborizing with the thoracoacromial cutaneous branch in the deltoid region. Delay procedures can help capture more distal extensions supplied by angiosomes of the subscapular and circumflex humeral vessels. The flap has largely been superceded by thinner and more pliable free fasciocutaneous flaps (radial forearm and anterior thigh).

9.9.8 Pectoralis Major Flap [9]

Ariyan described this musculocutaneous flap for head and neck reconstruction in 1979, whilst Arnold and Pairolero emphasised its uses in anterior chest wall (sternotomy) repair the same year. The triangular pectoralis major muscle, on the upper and front part of the chest arises from the sternum, clavicle and first five ribs, inserting as a tendon into the intertubercular groove of the humerus. Its vascular pedicle is deep to the muscle from the pectoral branch of the thoracoacromial axis (from the second part of the axillary artery). The surface landmark for this pedicle follows an oblique line from the coracoid process to the xiphisternum. The motor nerve supply is from the lateral pectoral nerve to the upper half and the medial pectoral nerve to the lower half of the muscle. This flap can be used as a pure muscle flap including a turn-over variant for sternotomy wounds, or as a musculocutaneous flap. Beware of RIMA and LIMA coronary artery donors.

9.9.9 Latissimus Dorsi Flap [10]

The original Latissimus flap was described by Tansini in 1906, derided by Halsted and rediscovered by Olivari in 1976. This large flat triangular muscle covering the lower back arises from the posterior iliac crest, sacrum, thoracolumbar vertebrae (T6–T12) plus ninth and tenth ribs, and inserts as a tendon behind pectoralis major in the intertubercular groove of the humerus. The dominant vascular pedicle, deep to the muscle is the thoracodorsal artery and vein, arising from the subscapular vessels, with a reverse option available on the lumbosacral perforators. The motor nerve supply is from the thoracodorsal nerve from the posterior cord of the brachial plexus. This flap is used in breast and chest wall reconstruction, upper limb reconstruction using a pedicled variant and lower limb reconstruction as a free flap.

In 50% of cases there is an angular branch to the lateral border of the scapular, making an osteo-myocutaneous variant possible.

9.9.10 Hand Flaps [11]

Multiple flaps have been described for hand reconstruction. These include Cross finger flaps of Gurdin et al. in 1950, First Dorsal Metacarpal Artery flap (FDMA) of Foucher in 1979, the Homodigital islanded finger flaps of Venkatswami (1980) and Evans (1988), and the dorsal hand flap of Quaba (1990). The FDMA arises from the lateral radial artery in the anatomical snuffbox and runs distally over the first dorsal interosseous muscle, terminating as the external dorsal artery of the index finger. Innervation is via the terminal branches of the superficial radial nerve. The dorsal hand flap is based on a direct branch of the dorsal metacarpal artery, which perforates just distal to the inter-tendinous connections of the extensor digitorum communis, or 5–10 mm proximal to the corresponding metacarpo-phalangeal joint. Cutaneous hand defects from trauma or cancer excision, with exposure of tendons, nerves or bone are the main indications for these innovative local flaps.

9.9.11 Forearm Flaps [12]

Yang et al. from China are credited with the first foreram flaps based on the radial artery for thumb reconstruction in 1978. Biemer in Germany learned these and inspired Soutar, Scheker, Tanner et al. from Glasgow to perform the first radial forearm free flap for retromolar trigone reconstruction in 1983. Lovie, Duncan and Glasson described the ulnar forearm free flap in 1984. The radial artery and venae comitantes are found in the lateral intermuscular septum of the forearm, distal to insertion of pronator teres and between FPL and FCR, with multiple branches supplying the adjacent flexor forearm muscles, distal radial border of the radius and overlying skin. The subcutaneous veins of the cephalic and basilic venous systems are usually incorporated. Antegrade or reverse flow options are available. The ulnar artery follows the ulnar nerve and can be used equally in similar fashion, but the radial artery must be intact and confirmed by the Allen flow test.

The ulnar artery in the proximal forearm is the segment distal to the common interosseous branch, which runs between FCU and FDS muscle bellies. Perforator branches are located here including a constant main fasciocutanous perforator 3–4 cm distal to the common interosseous branch. Both flaps provide thin pliable skin with or without a small segment of bone for reconstruction of the hand and/or the head and neck as a free flap.

9.9.12 Rectus Abdominis Flaps [13]

Interestingly, the free Transverse Rectus Abdominis Musculocutaneous (TRAM) flap was first performed by surgical trainees Fogdestam and Hamilton in 1978 whilst completing their anatomical studies in Gothenburg. The injection and dissection studies of the lower abdominal wall had started a year or two earlier when they were microvascular fellows in Melbourne. Holmström, who was an assistant at their two first clinical operations, subsequently published those cases omitting Fogdestam's and Hamilton's names.

Hartrampf, Scheflan and Black published the pedicled transverse abdominal island flap, some 4 years later in 1982. The paired rectus abdominis muscles arise from the pubic crest/tubercle and insert into the 5–7th costal cartilages. The dominant pedicle to the lower TRAM flap is via the perforators of the deep inferior epigastric vessels (DIEa, venae comitantes and superficial inferior epigastric vein). This has implications for the free perforator variants of the flap first published by Koshima in 1989 and popularised as the DIEP flaps by Blondeel et al. a decade later. Variants of the TRAM flap include the VRAM (vertical design) and ORAM (oblique design). The CT angiogram/venous phase as championed by Acosta et al. has refined the planning for perforator free flap breast reconstruction. Chest and pelvic/vaginal reconstruction are also good indications for rectus abdominis flaps.

9.9.13 Groin Flap [14]

McGregor and Jackson published the axial-patterned groin flap in 1972. It is based on the superficial circumflex iliac artery pedicle (SCIA) and venae comitantes. The main pedicle branches from the femoral artery in the groin traversing obliquely parallel to the inguinal ligament. Its point of origin is found as a landmark 2.5 cm inferior to the midpoint of a line from the anterior superior iliac spine (ASIS) to the pubic tubercle. The flap is raised laterally, superficial to the deep fascia until dissection reaches the lateral border of Sartorius, when the deep fascia should be included for safety. This flap's best clinical application is as a pedicled flap for covering hand and wrist defects, but requires a second stage about 4 weeks later.

Bilateral islanded groin flaps have been used for vaginal reconstruction and the classic bipedicled groin flap approach, is very safe in elective groin lymph node dissections.

The free groin flap has the disadvantage of a short vascular pedicle. Of all the flaps in the body, the groin flap has the least conspicuous donor site, being a fine linear scar.

9.9.14 Buttock Flaps [15]

Fujino described the gluteus maximus musculocutaneous flap in 1975. This large quadrilateral shaped muscle in the gluteal region has an extensive origin from the Ilium, Sacrum, Coccyx and their adjacent ligaments and fascia. It inserts in to the iliotibial tract of the fascia lata and the gluteal tuberosity of the femur. It has a double blood supply on its undersurface, the superior and inferior gluteal arteries. Its nerve supply is from the inferior gluteal nerve. When used as a large rotation flap it is the classical repair of sacral and ischial pressure sores.

9.9.15 Tensor Fascia Lata Flap [16]

Hill et al. described the free TFL in 1978. This muscle on the upper lateral aspect of the thigh has its origin from the iliac crest, anterior superior iliac spine and the deep surface of the fascia lata. It is inserted between the two layers of the iliotibial tract of the fascia lata. Its vascular supply is from the descending branch of the lateral circumflex femoral artery arising from the profunda femoral artery. Large venae comitantes accompany the artery as it enters the TFL muscle at the level of the greater trochanter, 10 cm inferior to the ASIS. Its nerve supply is from the superior gluteal nerve. Surgical uses of this flap include the repair of trochanteric and ischial pressure sores.

9.9.16 Gracilis Flap [17]

This was initially described as a musculocutaneous flap by Orticochea in 1972. The gracilis muscle is long and thin arising from the lower half of the body of the pubis and inserts into the medial surface of the upper tibia. Its main blood supply is the medial circumflex femoral artery arising from the profunda femoral artery and entering gracilis on its deep surface, at the junction of the upper quarter of the muscle with the lower three quarters. The obturator nerve (L1, L2) supplies the muscle, entering alongside the vascular pedicle after passing through the obturator foramen. The surface landmark of the anterior border of gracilis muscle is a line drawn from the pubic bone to the adductor tubercle of the femur. It can be used as a muscle or musculocutaneous flap, either on its vascular pedicle or as a free flap. The obturator artery branch to adductor longus should be preserved. Surgical uses include vaginal and perineal reconstruction and as a free muscle transfer.

9.9.17 Anterolateral Thigh Flap [18]

Song pioneered this flap in 1984. It is a large fascio-septocutaneous flap based on the cutaneous branch of the lateral circumflex femoral artery, which arises from the profunda femoral artery. The surface landmark for the perforator is a line drawn from the ASIS to the lateral edge of the patella bone, and the exact point is where the upper third of this line meets the middle third. The perforating cutaneous vessels emerge at the apex of the triangle formed by the confluence of rectus femoris, tensor fascia lata and vastus lateralis muscles.

It was originally used for trochanteric and ischial pressure sores but is now very popular as a free tissue transfer in head and neck reconstruction.

9.9.18 Posterior Thigh Flap [19]

Hurwitz described this cutaneous sliding flap in 1980. This is a triangular flap on the upper posterior aspect of the thigh. It is based on the end artery of the inferior gluteal artery which enters medially between the greater trochanter and ischium, deep to gluteus maximus and continuing vertically alongside the posterior cutaneous nerve of the thigh (S1–S3). The vascular territory extends as far distally as the popliteal fossa and it can be combined as a skin flap with the hamstring muscles. This flap is used to repair mid-sized pressure sores of the ischium and trochanteric regions. The flap is advanced upwards in to the defect and the donor repaired in V-Y fashion.

9.9.19 Reverse Sural Artery Flap [20]

Masquelet described this fasciocutaneous flap in 1992. This is a distally based fasciocutaneous or adipofascial flap on the midcalf. The superficial sural artery follows the course of the sural nerve and short saphenous vein of the posterolateral calf. The proximal vessel is found descending between the heads of gastrocnemius muscle, towards the ankle. Distal septocutaneous peroneal artery perforators approximately 5 cm above the lateral malleolus, capture the sural artery territory and allow for reverse flow. A skin island up to 9×6 cm can be planned and a 2.5 cm cuff of adipofascial tissue should be preserved around the pedicle. It is ideal for defects of the distal leg, ankle and foot.

9.9.20 Gastrocnemius Muscle Flaps [21]

Pers and Medgyesi are referenced as early pioneers of these calf muscle flaps in 1973. The pedicles are the lateral and medial sural branches of the popliteal artery and accompanying venae comitantes. The motor nerves are branches of the tibial nerve. The neurovascular pedicles enter the gastrocnemius muscles on their deep surfaces. The medial head of gastrocnemius is the larger flap of the two. Surgical uses include the inferior thigh, knee and lower extremity.

9.9.21 Extensor Digitorum Brevis Muscle Flap [22]

Barfred and Reumert described this flap in 1973.

This is a small multipennate muscle arising from the lateral aspect of the calcaneum and lying obliquely under the extensor digitorum longus tendons to the toes. The lateral tarsal branch of the dorsalis pedis artery is the dominant vascular pedicle, found just distal to the extensor retinaculum. It enters the muscle deeply and is accompanied by venae comitantes which drain into the anterior tibial vein. Surgical uses of this muscle flap include small skin defects of the distal leg, ankle and foot.

9.9.22 Medial Plantar Flap [23]

Morrison described this fasciocutaneous flap on the medial, non-weight-bearing side of the foot in 1983. It provides glabrous skin supplied by perforators from the medial plantar branch of the posterior tibial artery deep to abductor hallucis muscle. The skin island is raised distal to proximal, off the flexor hallucis brevis and just deep to the neurovascular plane. The cutaneous fascicle bundles of the medial plantar nerve can be carefully preserved to retain sensation in the flap. This requires an interneural dissection under tourniquet and with magnification. The distal branches of the medial plantar nerve are preserved. Surgical uses include heel reconstruction as a pedicled flap and for the contralateral heel as a free flap.

References

1. Acland's DVD Atlas of human anatomy Vol. 1 – 5, Lippincott?
2. Holmes AD, Marshall KA. Uses of the temporalis muscle flap in blanking out orbits. Plast Reconstr Surg. 1979;63:336.
3. Burget GC, Menick FJ. The paramedian forehead flap, aesthetic reconstruction of the nose (Mosby), Chap. 2; 1994, p. 57–91.
4. Pribaz JJ, et al. A new intraoral flap: facial artery musculomucosal (FAMM) flap. Plast Reconstr Surg. 1992;90(3):421–9.
5. Kaplan I, Goldwyn RM. The versatility of the laterally based cervicofacial flap for cheek repairs. Plast Reconstr Surg. 1978;61(3):390–3.
6. Lamberty BG. The supra-clavicular axial patterned flap. Br J Plast Surg. 1979;32:207–12.

7. McCraw JB, Magee WP, Kalwaic H. Uses of the trapezius and sternomastoid myocutaneous flaps in head and neck reconstruction. Plast Reconstr Surg. 1979;63:49.
8. Brown GED. The indirect deltopectotal flap. Br J Plast Surg. 1976;29:122–5.
9. Arnold PG, Pailero PC. Use of pectoralis major muscle flaps to repair defects of anterior chest wall. Plast Reconstr Surg. 1979;63(2):201–13.
10. Olivari N. The latissimus flap. Br J Plast Surg. 1976;29:126.
11. Quaba AA, Davison PM. The distally-based Doral hand flap. Br J Plast Surg. 1990;43:28.
12. Soutar DS, Tanner NSB. The radial forearm flap in the management of soft tissue injuries of the hand. Br J Plast Surg. 1984;37:18.
13. Hartrampf CR, Scheflan M, Black PW. Breast reconstruction with a transverse abdominal island flap. Plast Reconstr Surg. 1982;69:216.
14. Moschella F, Cordova A. Vaginal reconstruction with bilateral island extended groin flaps: description of a personal technique. Plast Reconstr Surg. 1994;7:1079–84.
15. Yanai A, Kosaka Y, Teraoka A. Several types of gluteus maximus musculocutaneous flaps for closure of sacral decubitus ulcer – refinements on design. Eur J Plast Surg. 1991;14:157–63.
16. Hill HL, et al. The tensor fascia lata myocutaneous free flap. Plast Reconstr Surg. 1978;61:517–22.
17. Mathes SJ, Nahai F. Reconstructive surgery: principles, anatomy & technique. Section 12B; 1997, p. 1173–91.
18. Neligan PC, Lannon DA. Versatility of the pedicled anterolateral thigh flap. Clin Plast Surg. 2010;37:677–81.
19. Lüscher NJ. Decubitus ulcers of the pelvic region – diagnosis & surgical therapy. Cambridge: Hogrefe & Huber Publishers; 1992. p. 116–9.
20. Mahboub T, Gad M. Increasing versatility of reverse-flow sural flap in distal leg & foot reconstruction. Egypt J Plast Reconstr Surg. 2004;28(92):99–112.
21. Pers M, Medgyesi S. Pedicle muscle flaps and their applications in surgery of repair. Br J Plast Surg. 1973;26:313.
22. Giordano PA, Argenson C, Pequignot JP. Extensor digitorum brevis as an island flap in reconstruction of soft tissues in the lower limb. Plast Reconstr Surg. 1989;83:100–9.
23. Morrison WA, et al. The instep of the foot as a fasciocutaneous island and as a free flap for heel defects. Plast Reconstr Surg. 1983;72:56–63.

Anaesthesia for Plastic Surgeons

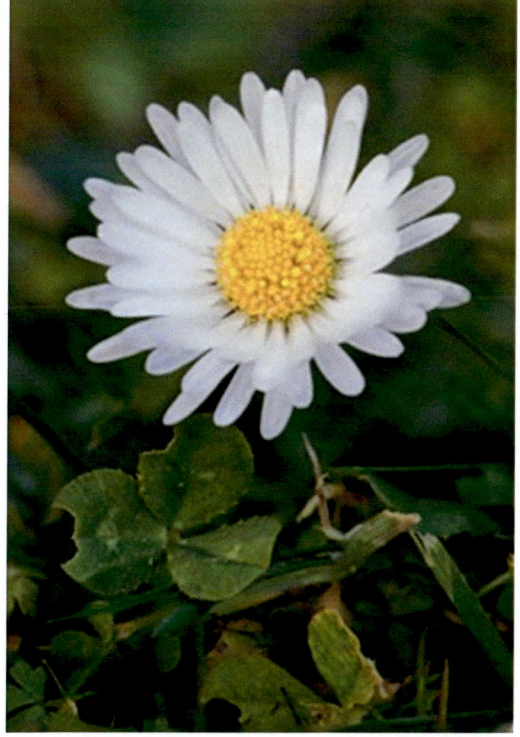

Daisy

The thin line between life and death

(Dr David Galler 2016)

Drs. Sophie Klaassen and Katherine Lanigan contributed significantly to this chapter.

© Springer Nature Singapore Pte Ltd. 2018
M. F. Klaassen and E. Brown, *An Examiner's Guide to Professional
Plastic Surgery Exams*, https://doi.org/10.1007/978-981-13-0689-1_10

10.1   Evolution of Plastic Surgery and Anaesthesia

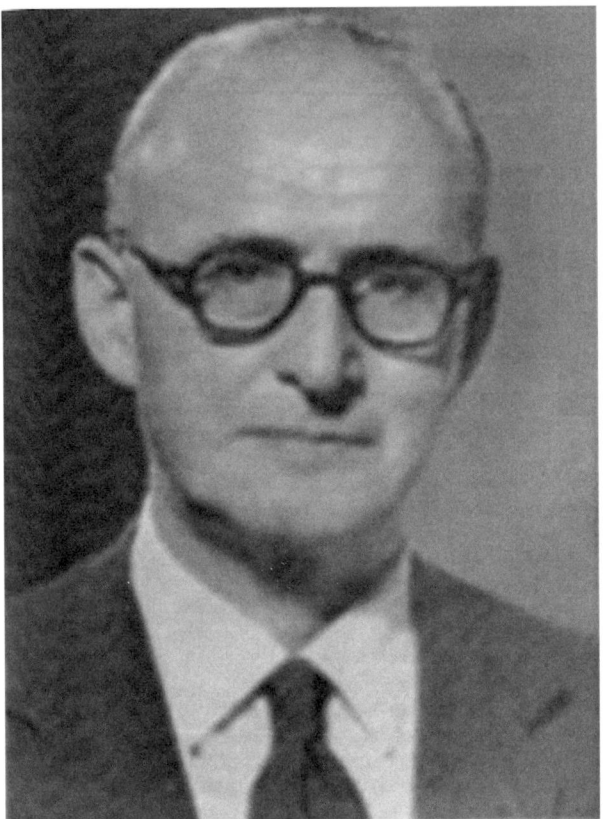

Ivan Whiteside Magill

It is significant and timely that the two specialties of anaesthesia and reconstructive plastic and maxillofacial surgery had their modern origins alongside each other at The Queens Hospital, Sidcup, Kent during the second half of the First World War (1916–1918). Major Harold Gillies with the support of the military hierarchy, a generous donation from Queen Mary and other private sponsorship established a purpose-built surgical hospital for facial and jaw injuries. His vision and goal was to bring all the selected facial injuries and the medical/nursing teams treating them to one specialist centre. British, Canadian, Australian and New Zealand divisions were working together, often with a friendly competitive edge and supported by multidisciplinary teams including anaesthetists, dental technicians, sculptors/artists and of course a dedicated nursing team. The anaesthetists were led by Captain R. Wade, who contributed to the 1920 book *Plastic Surgery of the Face* with six pages of remarks on anaesthesia. Later Captain Ivan Magill, an Ulsterman developed the first endotracheal tube at Sidcup to secure the airway of patients requiring complex facial reconstruction. The Magill forceps bear his name today.

10.2   Modern Surgeon/Anaesthetist Interactions

The skilful and expert delivery of peri-operative anaesthesia, monitoring of vital organs, fine-tuning of human physiology and pain management enable surgeons to achieve remarkable results without having to worry about the overall condition of the patient.

Successful surgery depends on a trilogy of anaesthetists (and their technicians), skilled operating room and ward nurses and surgeons (with their assistants).

The relationship between these health professionals is based on trust, respect, communication and teamwork.

The anaesthetic/surgeon/nursing team is a partnership and a professional working alliance that knows only too well, the sage words of Dr. David Galler (Senior Intensive Care Specialist, Middlemore)—*'the thin line between life and death'*.

I tell my patients that the anaesthetist caring for them and managing their anaesthetic during the operative procedure is the most important team member in the operating room (O.R.) … but collectively the medical team is all-important. The key factors for sophisticated and highly-developed anaesthetic surgical care are communication, situation awareness and clinical decision-making. The communication requires disclosure at a number of key periods in the surgical management:

1. Pre-operatively
2. Intra and peri-operatively
3. Post-operatively
4. Clinical audit and quality assurance

10.3   Pre-Operation

Diagnosis, considered options and definitive surgical plan must also address the co-morbidities, past medical history (including previous anaesthetic events, family history of drug allergies) and current medications which all contribute to the anaesthetic risk. The American Society of Anesthesiology (ASA) Physical Status (PS) Classification System developed by the American Society of Anesthesiologists (latest update, 2014) is summarised below.

ASA PS classification	Definition	Examples
ASA 1	A normal healthy patient	Healthy, non-smoking, no alcohol
ASA 2	Mild systemic disease	Mild disease without functional limitations (current smoker, social alcohol drinker, pregnancy, obesity (30 < BMI < 40), well-controlled diabetes mellitus/hypertension, mild lung disease)

(continued)

(continued)

ASA PS classification	Definition	Examples
ASA 3	Severe systemic disease	Substantive functional limitations—poorly controlled diabetes mellitus or hypertension, COPD, morbid obesity (BMI > 40), active hepatitis, alcohol dependence or abuse, implanted cardiac pacemaker, moderate reduction of ejection fraction with or without cardiac failure, End Stage Renal Disease (ESRD) undergoing regularly scheduled dialysis, premature infant <60 weeks, history (>3 months) of MI, CVA, TIA or CAD/stents
ASA 4	Severe systemic disease that is a threat to life	Recent (<3 months) MI, CVA, TIA or CAD/stents, ongoing cardiac ischaemia or severe valve dysfunction, severe reduction of ejection fraction, sepsis, DIC, ARD or ESRD not undergoing regularly scheduled dialysis
ASA 5	Moribund patient, not expected to survive without operation	Ruptured abdominal/thoracic aneurysm, massive trauma, intracranial bleed with mass effect, ischaemic bowel in the face of significant cardiac pathology or multiple organ/system dysfunction
ASA 6	Brain-dead patient whose organs are being removed for donor purposes	

The addition of 'E' denotes Emergency surgery.

e.g. ASA 2E.

In selected cases a pre-anaesthetic consult is required to address specific cardiovascular, respiratory and peri-anaesthetic risk factors. I generally send my anaesthetists a copy of my initial surgical report alerting them to a potential case and highlighting any obvious risk factors. This gives them time to arrange a workup specific to that individual patient. Recently we had a young woman with Ehlers-Danlos syndrome requiring major surgery and the workup required consultant anaesthetist and cardiologist involvement with echocardiography and other pre-surgery investigations. The early communication with your anaesthetic colleague is professionally appropriate, buys time and helps with the decisions about the most appropriate surgical facility for the case (outpatient, inpatient with or without ICU support).

10.4   Pre-Operative/Intra-Operative

The sequence of complex events, risk management and decision-making that occur during the surgical procedure are governed by all the modern strategies of communication skills, situation awareness, leadership, experience, clinical intuition and the sometimes urgent performance of practised emergency steps and manoeuvres. The realities of the very dangerous practice of surgery and anaesthesia require the full range of human factors and the familiarity of working within a team of known and experience colleagues. The older I get as a surgeon, the more I value this environment of trust and shared history of working relationships, because it instils quiet confidence. This is the best environment for our patients as well. It is not critical, because trained professionals following common non-technical strategies in the theatre should be able to work with each other without familiarity. The ideal is not always logistically possible for team selection.

10.5   Shared Airway

In certain surgeries involving the aerodigestive tract and head and neck surgery, the shared airway concept is in play. This is particularly an intraoperative scenario with rhinoplasty, intraoral surgery, orthognathic surgery and craniofacial surgery. The anaesthetist may have limited access to the patient's airway during the surgical procedure. Where such a situation is envisaged, the anaesthetist needs to be forewarned, so that the most appropriate anaesthetic and flexible airway conduits (endotracheal tubes, flexible laryngeal mask airway, elective tracheostomy) can be chosen.

10.6   Post-Operative

Sir Harold Gillies stated that the aftercare is as important as the planning and the execution of the surgery itself. This rings true for the post-anaesthetic care as well, in terms of immediate recovery, step-down to later recovery and recovery over the succeeding days, weeks and months. Following surgery and a general anaesthetic, most patients have a feeling of tiredness and reduced intellectual function. This can vary between patients and procedures. As a generalisation, for every hour of anaesthesia, I tell my patients it will take at least a week to fully recover their energy and intellectual function. This is important for patients to know, so that they can plan their elective surgery around their physical and intellectual commitments, such as sporting events and student examinations.

10.7   Local Anaesthetic

Local anaesthetic drugs are either Amino Esters or Amino Amides. Their method of action is to *block* action potentials in the nerve cell membrane. The nerve impulses are not propagated along the membrane and depolarization and repolarisation cannot proceed. Skin anaesthesia results and sometimes the nearby motor nerves are also blocked, causing temporary muscle weakness, e.g. brow ptosis and facial asymmetry.

The Amino Esters include Procaine and Cocaine. The Amino Amides include Lidocaine (TMXylocaine), Bupivacaine (TMMarcaine) and Ropivacaine (TMNaropin).

10.8   Maximum Safe Doses

Drug	Plain	With adrenaline	Duration	Onset time
Lidocaine	3–4 mg/kg	5–7 mg/kg	Medium	Quick
Bupivacaine	2.5 mg/kg	2.5 mg/kg	Long	Moderate
Ropivacaine	3–4 mg/kg	3–4 mg/kg	Long	Moderate

Lidocaine has a rapid onset of anaesthesia whilst Ropivacaine is characterised by slow onset of action and longevity. Lignocaine with Adrenaline and Ropivacaine can be combined to gain the benefits of both rapid onset and longevity of action. Remember that the collective dose is combined so safest to use 50% of the safe dose of the first local anaesthetic and no more than 50% of the second local anaesthetic.

Lidocaine has a rapid onset of anaesthesia whilst Ropivacaine is characterised by slow onset and prolonged duration of action.

10.9   Toxicity

Monitoring during local anaesthetic procedures is important for patient safety.

We suggest routine use of pulse meter or pulse oximeter.

Marcaine is the most toxic local anaesthetic potentially and has the highest lipid solubility. Cardiotoxicity from Marcaine overdose is almost always fatal and intravenous Intralipid 20% in the dose of 1.5 mL/kg stat over 60 seconds by infusion at 0.25 mL/kg/min is recommended as CPR continues. Naropin is the safest local anaesthetic in my experience and has a bonus vasoconstrictor affect, independent of adrenaline.

The earliest signs of local anaesthetic toxicity are CNS signs with cerebral excitation, restlessness, tinnitus, perioral tingling and light headedness followed progressively by seizures, loss of consciousness and eventually death, if not treated with emergency resuscitation. The ABCD of cardiac arrest management is initiated with Oxygen, airway and circulation support. Cardiovascular toxicity includes: hypotension, conduction blockade and cardiac arrest. Marcaine is associated with the highest risk of severe cardiac dysrhythmias and irreversible cardiovascular collapse.

10.10   ABCDE Management

Airway.
Breathing.
Circulation.
Disability (GCS: Glasgow Coma Score).
Exposure.

10.11   Cardiac Arrest During a Local Anaesthetic Procedure

When cardiac arrest is suspected, immediate cardiopulmonary resuscitation is critical to maintain oxygenation of vital organs. A vaso-vagal event can lead to pulselessness for a short period of time [1].

Send for urgent help.

Commence ABCDE with a cycle of 30 chest compressions, followed by two rescue breaths and then further compressions.

The first 2 min of proper CPR will give your patient 8 min more chance of survival.

Establishment of an airway with an endotracheal tube and administration of Oxygen.

Should circulation NOT be established, defibrillation should be initiated.

10.12   Safety Guidelines for Management of Severe LA Toxicity

1. *Recognition*
   Signs: sudden alteration in mental status, severe agitation or loss of consciousness with or without tonic-clonic convulsion. Cardiovascular collapse: sinus bradycardia, conduction blocks, asystole and ventricular tachyarrhythmias.
2. *Immediate management*
   Stop injecting. Call for help. Maintain airway, secure with an endotracheal tube. Give 100% oxygen and ensure adequate lung ventilation. Establish intravenous access. Control seizures with a benzodiazepam, thiopental or propofol in small incremental doses. Assess cardiovascular status throughout.
3. *Treatment*
   In Circulatory Arrest: start CPR, manage arrhythmias. Give Intravenous Lipid Emulsion (20% Lipid emulsion bolus 1.5 mL/kg over 1 min, start an IV infusion of 20% lipid emulsion at 15 mL/kg/h). After 5 min can give a maximum of two repeat boluses (same dose), 5 min between boluses. Continue infusion at same rate but Double rate to 30 mL/kg/h after 5 min.

   Without Circulatory Arrest: treat hypotension, bradycardia and tachyarrhythmias. Consider intravenous lipid emulsion.
4. *Follow-up*
   Arrange safe transfer to a clinical area with appropriate equipment for recovery of patient Post Anaesthesia Care Unit (PACU). Exclude pancreatitis by regular clinical review, including daily Amylase or Lipase assays for 2 days. Report case to national safety agency.

10.13   Different Types of Anaesthesia

General anaesthesia.
Local anaesthesia.
Regional anaesthesia.

Procedural sedation.

Conscious sedation.

Analgesia.

10.14 Guidelines for the Management of Postoperative Nausea and Vomiting (PONV)

(endorsed by Australian and New Zealand College of Anaesthetists)

Incidence of nausea is 50% and of vomiting is about 30%. Postoperative nausea and vomiting prophylaxis is therefore important. There is a subset of high risk patients. Risk factors include: females, <50 years, history of PONV, opioid use in PACU and nausea in PACU. The most likely causes of PONV are volatile anaesthetics, nitrous oxide and postoperative opioids. Strategies to reduce the risk of PONV include: avoidance of GA by using Regional Anaesthetic (in adults and children), use of propofol for induction and maintenance of anaesthesia, avoidance of nitrous oxide and volatile anaesthetics, minimization of intraoperative and postoperative opioids and adequate hydration.

Prophylaxis for PONV: this is reserved for patients who are at high risk of PONV and the evidence from multiple literature studies is that combination therapy (multimodal approach) is best.

For Adults pharmacologic combinations include:

Droperidol + dexamethasone.

5-HT3 receptor antagonist + dexamethasone.

5-HT3 receptor antagonist + droperidol.

5-HT3 receptor antagonist + dexamethasone + droperidol.

Ondansetron + casopitant.

For Children pharmacologic combinations include:

Ondansetron 0.05 mg/kg + dexamethasone 0.015 mg/kg.

Ondansetron 0.1 mg/kg + droperidol 0.015 mg/kg.

Tropisetron 0.1 mg/kg + dexamethasone 0.5 mg/kg.

All of the above drugs have potential side effects.

When nausea and vomiting occur postoperatively, treatment should be administered with an antiemetic from a pharmacologic class that is different from the prophylactic drug initially given [2].

10.15 Anaesthetic Emergencies/Critical Events

1. Can't intubate can't oxygenate (CICO)
2. Emergency tracheostomy
3. Anaphylaxis in the operating theatre
4. Malignant hyperthermia in the operating theatre
5. Fire in the operating theatre

10.16 Can't Intubate Can't Oxygenate (CICO)

CICO arises when attempts to manage the airway by tracheal intubation, face-mask ventilation, or placement of a supraglottic airway device have all failed. Hypoxic brain damage and death will result unless there is a rapid resolution. This is an emergency. Rehearsed protocols should be initiated early and surgical airway access achieved with either a mini-tracheotomy or an emergency tracheostomy [3].

10.17 Emergency Tracheostomy

Midline incision inferior to the cricoid cartilage (4–5 cm long), dissect between and retract the strap muscles laterally. Identify the tracheal rings and make either a cruciate incision or Bjork cartilage flap and introduce the tracheostomy tube for connection to the Oxygen supply and ventilation system. When the first sign of CI (Can't Intubate) is defined, call for tracheostomy set.

10.18 Anaphylaxis

Anaphylaxis during anaesthesia can present as cardiovascular collapse, airway obstruction, and/or skin manifestations.

Usual suspects include: neuromuscular blocking agents, natural rubber latex, antibiotics, plasma volume expanders, IV anaesthetic drugs and Betadine.

10.19 Management of Patient with Suspected Anaphylaxis During Anaesthesia:

1. Stop administration of all agents likely to have caused the anaphylaxis.
2. Call for help.
3. Maintain airway, give 100% oxygen and lie patient flat with legs elevated.
4. Give epinephrine (adrenaline). This may be given intramuscularly in a dose of 0.5–1 mg (0.5–1 mL of 1:1000) and may be repeated every 10 min according to the arterial pressure and pulse until improvement occurs. Alternatively, 50–100 μg intravenously (0.5–1 mL of 1:10,000) over 1 min has been recommended for hypotension with titration of further doses as required.

Secondary therapy

1. Give antihistamines (chlorpheniramine 10–20 mg by slow intravenous infusion).
2. Give corticosteroids (100–500 mg hydrocortisone slowly iv).
3. Bronchodilators may be required for persistent bronchospasm.

10.20 Malignant Hyperthermia (MH)

This is a rare pharmacogenetic disorder. It is fatal if prompt treatment is not instituted. Multiple high priority tasks must be attended to simultaneously and Resource Kits are available in all theatres and a laminated MH double-sided A4 sized *MH Crisis Initial Management Card* should be attached to each anaesthetic machine.

The most senior anaesthetist should co-ordinate crisis management;

1. Declare Emergency
2. Call for HELP
3. Send for MH box and supplies
4. Turn off volatile agent and remove vaporises from anaesthetic machine
5. Hyperventilate with 100% oxygen at >15 L/min
6. Commence IV anaesthesia maintenance (e.g. Propofol infusion)
7. *Dantrolene administration is the priority*

Signs and symptoms of MH.
Masseter spasm after Suxamethonium.
Tachypnoea and raised end tidal carbon dioxide.
Tachycardia.
Cardiac arrhythmias.
Rapid rise in temperature.
Respiratory and metabolic acidosis.
Hyperkalaemia.
Profuse sweating.
Cardiovascular instability.
Decreased Sp02 (peripheral capillary oxygen saturation) or mottling of skin.
Generalised muscular rigidity.
Myoglobinuria (dark-coloured urine).
Generalised muscle ache (awake patient).
Grossly raised serum CK.
Coagulopathy.
Cardiac Arrest.

10.21 Fires in the Operating Room

Involving patient.
As part of a building fire.
Chemical burns.

These can be either airway or non-airway fires. Fire is always a risk in the operating theatre when there exists the 'fire triad' of oxidizer, ignition and fuel. The emergency management of an airway fire includes: stopping the procedure, removing the tracheal tube, stopping the flow of all airway gases and saline irrigation of the airway, saline irrigation of the airway. Once fire is extinguished the ventilation of the patient is re-established with the circuit or a self-inflating resuscitation bag. Ventilate with room air. Consider bronchoscopy and airway examination to remove tracheal fragments and other debris. Continue an ongoing management plan for the patient's damaged airway.

References

1. Thim T, Krarup NHV, Grove EL, Rohde CV, Løfgren B. Initial assessment and treatment with the Airway, Breathing, Circulation, Disability, Exposure (ABCDE) approach. Int J Gen Med. 2012;5:117–21. Published online 2012 Jan 31. https://doi.org/10.2147/IJGM.S28478.
2. Gan TJ, et al. Consensus guidelines for the management of postoperative nausea and vomiting. Anesth Analg. 2014;118(1):85–113.
3. Pracy JP, Brennan L, Cook TM, Hartle AJ, Marks RJ, McGrath BA, Narula A, Patel A. Surgical intervention during a Can't intubate Can't oxygenate (CICO) event: Emergency Front-of-neck Airway (FONA)? Br J Anaesth. 2016;117(4):426–8. https://doi.org/10.1093/bja/aew221. Published:19 September 2016.

Aesthetic Surgery Principles

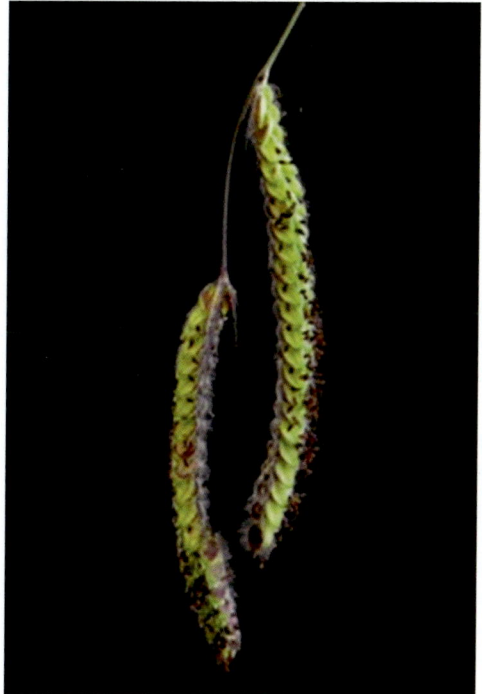

Paspalum

Plastic surgery requires skills in both reconstructive and cosmetic surgery.
Reconstructive surgery has a goal to restore the normal.
Cosmetic surgery aims to surpass the normal.
No-one can call themselves a plastic surgeon unless they are competent at both reconstructive and cosmetic surgery.

(Sir Harold Delf Gillies)

© Springer Nature Singapore Pte Ltd. 2018
M. F. Klaassen and E. Brown, *An Examiner's Guide to Professional Plastic Surgery Exams*, https://doi.org/10.1007/978-981-13-0689-1_11

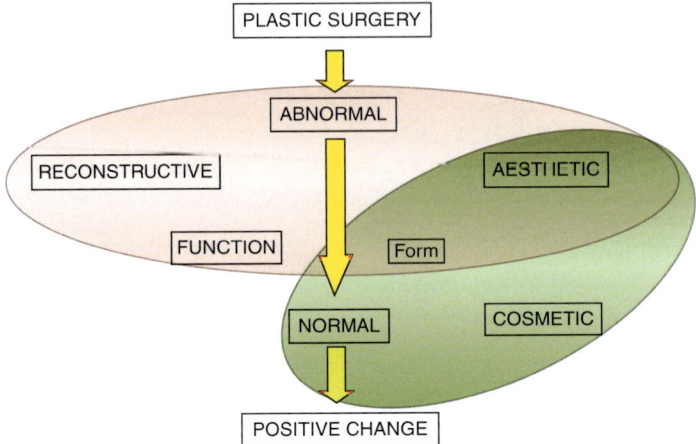

Fig. 11.1 Differences between reconstructive and cosmetic plastic surgery [1]

Professor Andrew Burd, former Chief and Professor, Division of Plastic, Reconstructive and Aesthetic Surgery, Department of Surgery, Chinese University of Hong Kong and Prince of Wales Hospital, re-emphasised the principle of Gillies regarding aesthetic surgery.

He illustrated this in his 2008 paper on the differences and balance between reconstructive and aesthetic surgery from an educational and training perspective with a very helpful Venn diagram (Fig. 11.1).

This Venn diagram indicates the essential difference between Reconstructive Plastic Surgery and Cosmetic Plastic Surgery and complements the above quotation of Harold Gillies.

Both are based on similar Aesthetic Principles. The Reconstructive patient presents with some abnormality that requires correction.

The Cosmetic patient presents essentially within the range of normality and wishes their features to be enhanced.

This paper was written to stem the growing tide of misrepresentation of plastic surgeons being almost exclusively associated with cosmetic surgery.

Burd articulates this even more clearly when he writes 'aesthetic surgery principles include beauty, harmony, shape and form as well as the less tangible but equally functional equivalents of gracefulness and naturalness'.

One of Dr. Ralph Millard's principles reiterated this with 'Understand the beautiful normal'.

Plastic surgery had its origins in the theatres of war surgery, even before the challenges that The Great War (1914–1918) delivered. Is there anything less worthy than restoring a disfigured serviceman or woman with an aesthetic reconstruction, that allows them to rehabilitate and return to a productive and happy lifestyle? Should not a child's congenital cleft lip and palate deformity be restored to a form and function that acknowledges the beautiful normal and brings joy to the parents, grandparents and siblings.

I have come to understand some essential principles of aesthetic surgery after more than 30 years of active practice:

1. Your aesthetic surgery patient is not a client, but a patient.
2. Connectedness with your patient leads to a confident patient (McIndoe Principle).
3. The trust and confidence between surgeon and patient is bilateral.
4. Aesthetic surgery is real surgery with all the potential risks, hazards and complications.
5. Complications after aesthetic surgery require extraordinary attention and effort.
6. There is always an agenda for the patient requesting aesthetic improvement (Patrick Jerome Beehan Principle).
7. Aesthetic surgery is practised within a private practice setting so as well as a comprehensive informed consent there should be an equally comprehensive financial consent.
8. Always ask the patient whether they could cope with a complication and the added costs that this would potentially cause.
9. Use old photographs to study and predict the expected result from facial aesthetic surgery procedures.
10. Have an anatomist's knowledge of the applied anatomy and explain this in language the patient can understand. Crisalix virtual aesthetic software is useful tool in the modern age.
11. Don't operate on aesthetic patients with whom you cannot establish a friendly trusting relationship.
12. You will discover much about the patient's psyche after the surgery.
13. When first starting work as a specialist, keep the aesthetic surgery operations simple, safe and predictable.
14. Refer patients to more experienced colleagues when their expectations demand it.
15. Learn to say NO, and when the patient returns keep saying NO (John P. Bennett first Principle).
16. Never be a salesman/saleswoman (John P. Bennett 2nd Principle).
17. Document every conversation, phone call, photograph and always give the patient copies of their medical reports, operative notes and post-operative notes.
18. When you get into trouble, recognise this early and call for help (Brent Tanner Principle).
19. No one needs an aesthetic operation to save their life.
20. As a plastic surgeon you have the right to not perform cosmetic surgery, but you should know about it, its advantages, limitations and complications.
21. The improvement in a patient's self confidence and self-esteem when the aesthetic surgery is successful is profound.
22. Many patients moving forward may need to consider maintenance procedures and these should be selected carefully.

23. When a patient is unhappy and you have done the best you can then this is a BIG problem for both of you.
24. When the patient is happy but you think you didn't achieve your best, keep this thought to yourself.
25. Operate on friends and family at your peril.

> Improvement in the results of facelift surgery is achieved by clear understanding of the anatomy of the deformity of facial aging and application of the appropriate procedure.
>
> (Jack Q. Owsley, 1983) [2]

11.1   Some Common Aesthetic Surgery Procedures

Hair replacement	Skin resurfacing
Browlift	Labioplasty
Blepharoplasty	
Facelift	
Necklift	
Otoplasty	
Rhinoplasty	
Facial implants	
Lipomorphoplasty	
Botox and fillers	
Breast augmentation	
Mastopexy	
Liposuction	
Gynaecomastia correction	
Body Contouring Surgery	
Abdominoplasty	
Buttock and thigh lift	
Brachioplasty	

References

1. Burd A. Plastic, reconstructive & aesthetic surgery. Med Bull. 2008;13(7):25–7.
2. Owsley JQ. Aesthetic facial surgery. Philadelphia: W.B. Saunders Company; 1994.

Science Principles for Plastic Surgery 12

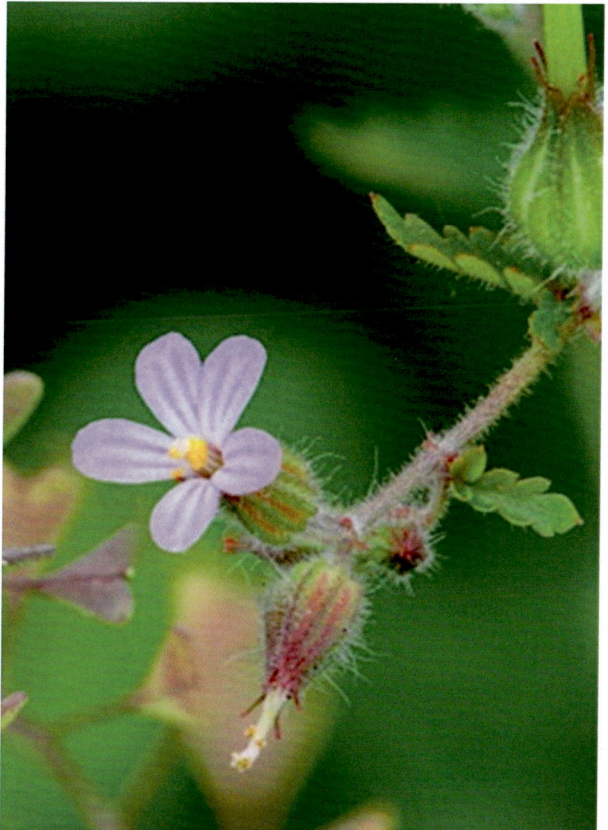

Geranium purpureum

© Springer Nature Singapore Pte Ltd. 2018
M. F. Klaassen and E. Brown, *An Examiner's Guide to Professional Plastic Surgery Exams*, https://doi.org/10.1007/978-981-13-0689-1_12

Science is a way of thinking much more than it is a body of knowledge

(Carl Sagan)

The important thing is to never stop thinking

(Albert Einstein)

In support of the two famous quotes above, Sir Harold Delf Gillies once remarked that plastic surgery was a constant battle between beauty and blood supply. Beauty is something we should never stop thinking about as plastic surgeons, because it is everywhere we look for it and the beautiful normal in form, function and the human aesthetic is our goal. The blood supply to vital organs, bones, soft tissue integument and the skin are quintessentially what define plastic and reconstructive surgery as a science and a craft. Add to this mix the art and vision of an artist, together with good listening skills, compassion and connectedness of a good doctor; that is all you need.

12.1   Blood Supply of Skin

An understanding and appreciation of the circulatory system is mandatory for primary and secondary healing. Historically the pioneering work of Salmon et al. defined the anatomical basis of blood supply to the body. By modern standards this is an integrated network of vasculature coursing in a predictable pattern from named source arteries through muscles and fascia to the subdermal plexus and then in reverse through the venous tributaries back to the named source veins. The heart, that reliable, resilient and marvellous pump organ, is what drives it all [1].

William Harvey in 1628 defined the modern concept of blood supply.

Tomsa (1873), Manchot (1889) and Salmon (1936) were the early contributors to the understanding of the blood supply of the skin, by painstaking dissection and observation. Salmon from Paris introduced the classification of direct and indirect cutaneous arteries. The latter being the musculocutaneous, neurocutaneous and fasciocutaneous perforators, so important in today's local and loco-regional flaps. Salmon's writing considered the surgical implications and introduced the concept of cutaneous arterial territories, each with a certain autonomy. Many of these early publications were written in German or French and were not readily available to the English-speaking surgeons.

Gillies et al. found a practical if not altogether reliable way to close war wounds with random pattern flaps of a limited length to breadth ratio. Some authors have criticised this approach with a retrospective smugness, but we believe it simply a case of appreciating historical developments that have all contributed to the rich tapestry of plastic surgery concepts.

Taylor et al. confirmed the findings of Manchot and Salmon in the twentieth century and described the Angiosomes, a series of anatomical three-dimensional vascular territories. These are governed by reliable principles:

1. The connections between adjacent cutaneous arteries are either by true anastomoses, without change in caliber, or by reduced-caliber choke anastomotic vessels

2. One adjacent anatomical/cutaneous perforator territory (skin module) can be captured with safety radially in any direction on the perforator at the flap base.
3. Most muscles span two or more angiosomes and are supplied from each territory, one is able to capture the skin island from one angiosome via the muscle supply in the adjacent territory.
4. Vessels follow the connective tissue framework of the body.
5. Vessels radiate from fixed to mobile areas.
6. Vessels hitchhike with nerves.
7. Vessel size and orientation are a product of tissue growth and differentiation.

Vessels obey "The Law of Equilibrium" (If one vessel is small, its partner is large to compensate and vice versa.)

8. Vessels have a relatively constant destination but may have a variable origin.
9. The vessels form a continuous unbroken network.

The Angiotome concept closely matches the angiosome theory. Behan and Wilson started work on this in 1973 whilst research fellows in London. The *angiotome* is an area of skin that survives when cut as a flap, supplied by an axial vessel extended by its communication with branches from the adjacent vessel. The concept emphasises the role of the dermatome and the intrinsic neurocutaneous vascular supply of the human skin. This is essential to the planning of bespoke keystone perforator island flaps (KPIFs).

The fasciocutaneous island flaps that Behan was using to cover compound lower limb fractures in the 1990s developed into the keystone perforator island flaps. Serendipitously he combined the dermatome pattern of design with the concept of angiotome vascular perfusion.

Essentially a dermatome associated with somite development is an area of the skin supplied by a spinal nerve. If a spinal nerve is to develop from the notochord (primitive streak area), it must have an arteriovenous support network for this autonomic-somatic neural complex. The basic embryological principle is confirmed. The neurovascular structures subsequently become arborized, which account for their distal perfusion from minute vascular links.

Lymphatic development must also accompany such arborisation with development and growth. This simple aide-memoire of a dermatomal link, based on a fascial support without skeletonizing the perforator source, allows the accompanying lymphatic and autonomic fibres to be retained.

Finally, there are humoural factors (nitrous oxide), which also operate within this scheme [2, 3].

12.2   Local Flap Principles

1. Elliptical excision and sliding flap repair is the basis of all traditional local flap repairs.

2. Limberg (1946) described as a paradox the principle that in order to close a skin defect, a nearby triangle of healthy skin equal in size to the defect is discarded.
3. Burow and Bernard both applied this principle to their triangular excisions.
4. Tension in a flap decreases the blood flow in the flap.
5. Even if this decreased flap blood flow is not enough to cause skin necrosis, atrophy will occur at a subcutaneous level, to produce a depressed scar at the distal end of the flap.
6. David Tolhurst (1988) described an Atomic System for classifying flaps where he compares all flap repairs to the nucleus and electrons of an atom.
7. The nucleus lists the tissue components of the flaps (e.g. skin, fat, fascia, muscle …).
8. The outer shell system lists the various flap characteristics (e.g. skin or non-skin blood supply, axial or random pattern, form, destination and special preparation).

12.3 Tolhurst's Atomic System for Classifying Flaps

Klaassen et al. Simply Local Flaps page 25, Fig. 12.1, Springer International Publishing AG 2017.

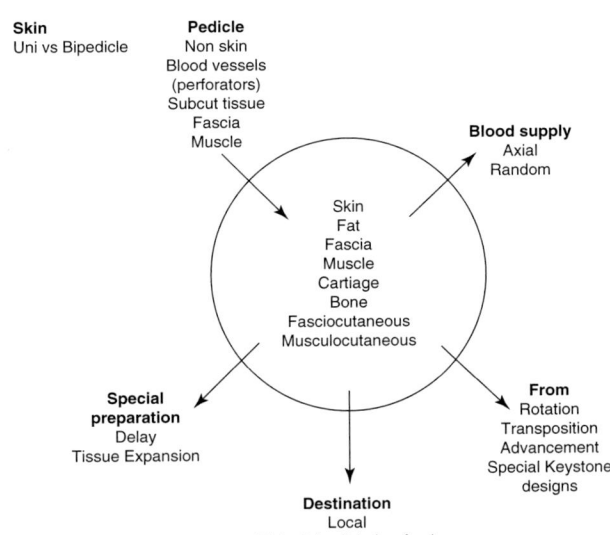

Fig. 12.1 The atomic system for classification of flaps by David Tolhurst (with his express permission)

12.4   Wound Healing

Wound healing involves a complex physiological process at a cellular level involving stem cells, inflammatory cells, matrix molecules, cytokines and various mediators. There are four distinct phases of healing:

1. Coagulation phase (immediate)
2. Inflammatory response phase (48–72 h)
3. Proliferative phase (days 4–21)
4. Maturation phase (up to 1 year)

The proliferative phase includes the formation of extracellular matrix (ECM), angiogenesis and re-epithelialisation. Fibrillar collagen is the main structural component of the ECM responsible for both elasticity and strength in an intact scar. Collagen type I and type III are recognised as the main building blocks of a scar and although type III increases more than type I in the early stages of healing, it decreases to normal levels during the final maturation stage.

12.5   Hypertrophic and Keloid Scars

Fibroblasts and diseased stem cell fibroblasts contribute to the clinical problems of hypertrophic and keloid scars. The spectrum from physiologically normal to keloid scar is a continuous one determined by genetically influenced control pathways involving apotosis, growth factors and angiogenesis. Fibroblasts transform into myofibroblastics which produce the collagen types I & III, cytokines and influence wound contraction. Various forms of collagenase and proteinase influence the final scar formation. Some patients have a propensity to develop hypertrophic scars. Those areas of the body that are prone to hypertrophic scars, are: anterior chest and deltoid regions.

12.6   Management Options for Hypertrophic and Keloid Scars (Mild—Severe)

Micropore tape compression (for 12 weeks).
   Silicone gel/sheeting.
   Intralesional corticosteroid/5FU/Interferon.
   Topical cryotherapy.
   Intralesional cryotherapy (Cryoshape probe)—*the most efficacious.*

LASER ablation.

Surgery + immediate radiation.

12.7   Surgical Site Infection

Exam candidates should have a full appreciation of the implications of Surgical Site Infection and be prepared for infection related questions.

We recommend you be familiar with recent published reports and recommend the 2017 Wisconsin Division of Public Health Supplemental Guidance for the Prevention of Surgical Site Infections: An Evidence-Based Perspective [4].

The Core Section describes recommendations that should be applied to all surgical procedures.

The candidate should be familiar with:

The size and evidence for the problem

Antibiotic prophylaxis

Glycaemic control

Normothermia

Oxygenation

Skin prep with alcohol-based antiseptics

Potential risk with administration of blood products during arthroplasty surgery

The role of Microbiol biofilms.

12.8   Skin Microbiology

There is a balance between normal skin flora and innate immunity. 90% of the resident aerobic skin flora is *Staphylococcus epidermidis*. It is generally regarded as a commensal but it can also act as a pathogen. *Staphylococcus aureus* is the most common pathogen isolated in surgical site infections.

$$\frac{\text{Dose of bacteria} \times \text{virulence}}{\text{Resistance of the host}} = \text{Risk of Surgical Site Infection}$$

The equilibrium is broken.

Remember that severe inflammation can be sometimes mistaken for surgical site infection. This is particularly common with sutures used for local flaps that are left in-situ for more than 2 weeks.

The dose of bacteria is significant for inoculation. Dr. Martin Robson showed that the critical figure for infection is 10^6 organisms per gram of tissue [5].

12.9   Other Important Scientific Concepts

Primitive Streak the faint streak which is the earliest trace of the embryo in the fertilized ovum of a higher vertebrate.

Telomere a compound structure at the end of a chromosome.

Apoptosis the death of cells which occurs as a normal and controlled part of an organism's growth or development. Also called programmed cell death.

Atrophy (of body tissue or an organ) is a wasting away, especially as a result of the degeneration of cells, or becoming vestigial during evolution [6].

References

1. Galler D. Things that matter – stories of life and death. Crows Nest: Allen & Unwin; 2016.
2. Behan FC. The fasciocutaneous island flap: an extension of the angiotome concept. Aust NZ J Surg. 1992;62(11):874–86.
3. Behan FC. Fasciocutaneous island flaps for orthopaedic management in lower limb— reconstruction using dermatomal precincts. Aust NZ J Surg. 1994;64:155–66.
4. Edmiston CE et al. Wisconsin division of public health supplemental guidance for the prevention of surgical site infection: an evidence-based perspective Jan 2017 (Rev. 5/2017).
5. Robson MC. Wound infection. A failure of wound healing caused by an imbalance of bacteria. Surg Clin North Am. 1997;77:637–50.
6. Mokos ZB, Jović A, Grgurević L, Dumić-Čule I, Kostović K, Čeović R, Marinović B. Current therapeutic approach to hypertrophic scars. Front Med. 2017;4:83. https://doi.org/10.3389/fmed.2017.00083.

The Successful Candidate

Observable Features Deconstructed

13

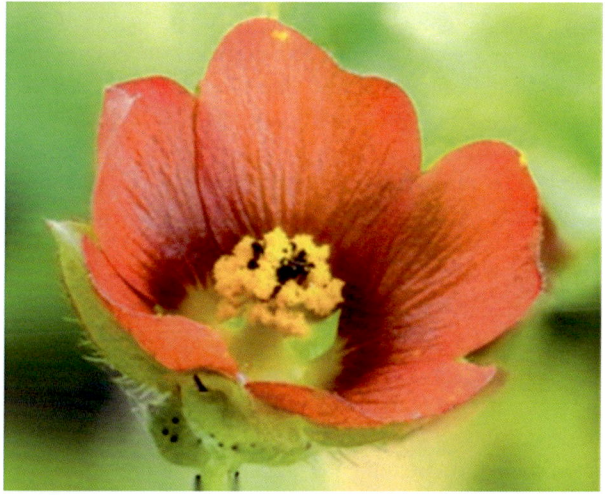

Modiola

Success is a journey, not a destination.
The doing is often more important than the outcome.

(Arthur Ashe)

Over more than 16 years of examining and coaching young plastic surgeons for their final fellowship exams we have been able to observe and define a profile for what is the successful candidate. It is an observation of trainees from all over Australia and New Zealand, but includes a large number of International Medical Graduates (IMGs). Many of these candidates are presenting for the first time, and

© Springer Nature Singapore Pte Ltd. 2018
M. F. Klaassen and E. Brown, *An Examiner's Guide to Professional Plastic Surgery Exams*, https://doi.org/10.1007/978-981-13-0689-1_13

some for repeat attempts. For most of them it is a time of performance anxiety. We are exposed to them at a time when they are saturated with knowledge and attempting to combine this knowledge with clinical experience, decision-making and communication. The journey to FRACS (Plast) is long and hard. Increasingly this journey is being influenced by changing workplace practice: reduced clinical exposure, reduced clinical performance, reduced levels of responsibility, reduced after hours on-call, increased numbers of unprepared candidates and increased numbers of candidates who ignore the advice of their supervisors, with regard to preparedness for the exam.

One way of practising the organisation of one's thoughts is in the new patient and follow-up clinics. Dictate the patient notes in a logical and thoughtful way, being concise and creating a word picture. A busy consultant should be able to quickly read these notes and get an accurate picture of the clinical situation.

The standard for the FRACS exam is achievable and is all about universal competence and capability. Over the years a number of candidates have impressed as certainties for a successful result in the exam. A great many others have not quite been up to the same standard but have used the time between the coaching courses and the exam (usually a month) to realign, re-set and fine-tune their performance. There is a small group who clearly are not quite ready and often lack insight into how far off the mark they are.

This chapter focuses on the key features of the successful candidate.

Overall, the successful candidate brings a quiet calmness to the exam room. There is a vibe of composure, cool collectedness and a presence of mind. Competence exudes from them in every thought, interpretation, decision and communication. Someone described as competent has the necessary knowledge and skill to fulfil a particular role—in this case the role of a new consultant plastic surgeon.

Another way to describe the 'successful candidate' profile is to recognise the signs that they are organised mentally and clinically. They are able to think on their feet, apply basic logic, common-sense and principles to the problem at hand. It may be a complex clinical situation, with variable contributing factors and perhaps even a problem they have not encountered before. The successful candidate is able to dispel any anxiety, stay focused and remain unflappable. Unfortunately, these are human behaviour skill-sets that few of us are born with—but they can be learned. The absolute secret to this challenge is to start thinking and communicating in this style from day one of your advanced surgical training. As has been observed before, the common observation of junior surgical trainees who have competed intensely for advanced surgical training positions; once selected they drift into a 'cruise control mode' for a couple of years. Success brings with it the danger of complacency. This is a commonly observed flaw.

The key features of the successful candidate are summarised:

1. Prepare for the journey towards final fellowship exam early.
2. Knowledge needs to be married to clinical experience.
3. Have self-belief and ability to think on your feet.
4. Develop a structured and logical way of thinking.

5. Expect to be challenged.
6. Don't be intimidated, learn to handle the pressure.
7. Keep it simple.
8. Stay positive and healthy in mind and body.
9. Develop resilience.
10. Focus on the patient's problem and their welfare.
11. Use all the evidence provided (e.g. images, radiology, laboratory results).
12. Keep your answers brief and precise.

The Failed Candidate

14

How to Regroup, Reassess and Fight Back to Success

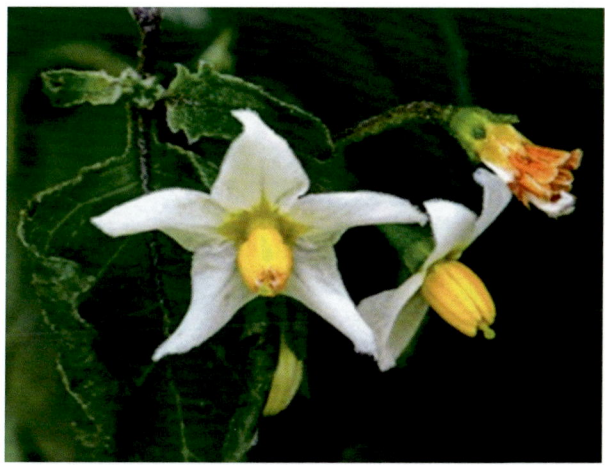

Solanum nigrum

Success is not final, failure is not fatal:
It is the courage to continue that counts.

(Winston Churchill)

For any consultant plastic surgeon who passed the final fellowship exam on their first attempt, they will not know if they did so with flying colours or by the skin of their teeth. The close marking system set by the Court of Examiners (RACS) is designed to be fair, transparent and defensible. After examining for several years, I know how close some candidates came to not crossing the line, but for them sweet success was the only reality.

© Springer Nature Singapore Pte Ltd. 2018
M. F. Klaassen and E. Brown, *An Examiner's Guide to Professional Plastic Surgery Exams*, https://doi.org/10.1007/978-981-13-0689-1_14

For the failed candidate, the reality is brutal and devastating. The decision that you are not yet ready, after years of training, study and toil is a bitter pill to swallow. 1988 and 1989 were not my finest years apart from the birth of our first son, because I was a failed candidate twice. For some years well into my appointment as a consultant plastic surgeon, nightmares of exam failure haunted me. This chapter is an attempt to get inside the mind of the failed candidate, to self-analyse and to try and find some patterns of failure that the well-prepared new candidate may find helpful. The other plastic surgeons who have shared their thoughts, experiences and reflections on failure before ultimate success, will remain anonymous but I am grateful and inspired by their courage. As Winston Churchill, that wonderfully gifted wordsmith and realist once said: 'Success consists of going from failure to failure without loss of enthusiasm'.

14.1   Candidate A (anonymous)

I attempted my first FRACS exam aged 32 years having completed 2 years of general surgery training, a year of surgical research and a year of orthopaedic training before 2 of 3 years of plastic surgery training. I was confident, had self-belief, seemed to be competent at the fundamental skills of plastic surgery and had been exposed to supervisors and mentors in two major teaching hospitals. I probably had not done quite enough textbook reading leading up to my first attempt, but had covered the syllabus and studied harder than I had ever done as an undergraduate medical student. I had two young children and responsibilities. It was important for me to progress with my plastic surgery career and overseas fellowship posts awaited.

In hindsight, I was over-confident and my attempts to 'bluff' through discussions with the experienced examiners was my undoing. I remember a particular short case, where a lateral tarsorrhaphy was required for the protection of the cornea in a patient with facial palsy. I had read about the temporary versus permanent tarsorrhaphy techniques, but never actually witnessed nor performed one myself. Instead of just defining the principles of tarsorraphy, I spoke with the confidence of a seasoned veteran and clearly was unconvincing. Another dark moment was when extolling the virtues of the McCash Open-Palm method for fasciectomy in Dupuytren's disease, for which I was very familiar but clearly one of the examiners did not favour this method. I did not have the situation awareness to change tack and offer alternative options, which clearly the examiner was searching for.

During the exam, the candidate has very little insight or feedback of their performance in the heat of the moment. The oral examinations seem to be over very quickly and examiners are trained to be impartial and neutral in their responses. Thirty years ago, when my contemporaries and I were preparing for the final fellowship exams, we knew very little about what to expect on the first attempt. This was before instructional videos, emails, internet or even cell phones. The clinical cases were a random selection of what each examiner brought to the table and there was no attempt at standardisation of the cases or the questions. Very few of the consultants had any interest in preparing the candidates for the exams. Earle Brown FRCS,

FRACS was for me an inspirational exception. He encouraged us to prepare in groups and gave up many hours of his personal time to coach us. I think he couldn't bear the thought of his senior registrar failing for a third time! The other annoying feature of the oral exams in Operative Surgery & Pathology in those early years was the presence of a general surgeon examiner, seconded to the plastic surgery mini-court. That often created difficulties and was a real threat to the candidates. I would love to see today how the general surgery mini-court would handle an experienced plastic surgeon examiner, challenging their candidates in part of the oral exam?

The failures hurt personally, especially my self-confidence, but in the long-term it made me stronger and gave me a self-belief that has endured for 30+ years. I am grateful to those who doubted me, because I am better for it. This has benefitted my patients too. Coping with this adversity makes you stronger and the resilience developed from facing disappointment, failure and bad news is a bonus. None of us know what tomorrow will bring, but we live in hope that it will be something better. Some days it will be grateful, healed and confident patients. Some days it will be wound complications, haematomas, lost flaps and grafts … with all the grief that is associated with these adverse events. Life as a surgeon requires passion, compassion, energy, self-belief, resilience and humility. When I look back at my surgical career now, I regret 'beating' myself up so much over a mere exam failure. It was a temporary setback, a hiccup on a long journey and in fact the benefits of having to cope with the failure far outweighed the detriments. Failure may temporarily bend you but ultimately it will strengthen you in more ways than you will ever appreciate. Failure can be turned into a bonus and a career asset. Over the years of teaching the next generation, my own experience of dealing with the failed exam has given me an insight and ability to help others. Their knowledge and competence is never in question, rather they need to find their self-belief and confidence again. It has given me enormous pleasure and pride to see a number of them ultimately succeed and this is always a reminder of how sweet success and triumph over adversity felt so long ago.

14.2   Candidate B

Thank you for the advice. I can only hope that I have recovered enough mentally, as it has been a pretty exhausting experience overall. I think I lost my composure on that first day of the exam. I was too nervous and wound up even before I started and that was a mistake. I knew the first day had gone badly—I had no confidence and was incredibly intimidated by my examiners. I made very bad decisions. In fact I probably went into the clinical vivas feeling fairly drained. I knew this was the wrong thing to do, but I perhaps pushed myself a bit too much in the weeks leading up to the exam. I did not achieve that study/relaxation balance and ignored the advice you had given: to stay fit and fresh going in. I will try to stay healthier and fitter next time round. Despite all the preparation and practice that I did with my mentors and colleagues, there is nothing that can really simulate the real exam.

14.2.1 Six Months Later …

I have passed my fellowship exam. Thank you for your encouragement & advice over the past few months. They have been difficult months, but in hindsight I have learnt a lot through the process of redoing this exam. Mainly about maintaining a healthy balance, looking after myself, and most importantly having confidence in my ability. It is such a mental game and if you do not have complete faith in yourself going in to the exam you have already lost the battle.

14.3   Candidate C

For me there are three phases to passing these exams after a disappointing run at it—all can be likened to 'bagging' a Munro (Scottish summit). Firstly you've got to recognise that you are in a 'valley'—let yourself wallow a bit and take a look around while you're down there—you don't want to be back in this place again. If you are really in deep and struggling to take the next step, you might actually need to talk to someone to help you get out. As a breed we're not used to failure, so it can hit harder. Get perspective from someone you respect.

Next is the ascent phase—where you take the familiar trudge up the side of the study mountain—but don't be complacent because you've been here before. Instead take the time to look at the view differently, notice new things, make the most of the second time going up because (it may be hard to hear right now), you will end up being better at what you do having had to make this climb a second time.

Finally, you have the actual summit (i.e. the exam). Take the feedback from the first time and make sure you never make these footing mistakes again. Have confidence in your muscle memory—you've been here before and that will take the edge off—though it will be no less exhilarating and adrenalin-charged. Mainly make sure you are determined and definite when you finally finish what you set out to do—because it's a long way down!

Some more specific advice I was given and some lessons I learnt about more effective study:

1. For the most part, the exam feedback is not that helpful. Read it once and file it.
2. Take a break. A proper break. Literally do not study or look at your notes for a month. Use this time to reconnect with your friends, family, get lots of exercise, indulge/eat out, break the routine. You need this to regroup and reenergize for round two.
3. Be critical and ruthless with who you spend time studying with. Every session must count to make you feel more confident or enhance your knowledge. It is about what you need, not what your study mates need. What works will be different for everyone—just don't compromise your own study for someone else's.

4. Don't be too proud to ask for time off, clinics, private sessions, etc.... ask your manager/supervisor of training to facilitate your need to attend cases, clinics to give you the confidence required for that particular topic, etc. (There will be time to repay the debt later).

5. Swap out of your on-calls. Your junior colleagues will get their turn later, you will have done your pay-it-forward. Ask for help and take it.

6. Be honest about productivity when studying. If it is not working go for a walk for half an hour and come back refreshed.

7. Early nights, healthy diet, restricted caffeine are all relevant to get the tortoise ready. You can't sprint like a hare for this exam, so look after yourself.

8. Spend time with your family/friends (people who like you!) each day. Find someone who is happy to hear the 'daily download', i.e. get the day out of your head so you can focus.

9. The reality is that you have to put; your life on hold to get this done. Your relationships. The things that matter to you. In the grand scheme of things this is just a small period of time when you have no choice but to be selfish—those people who matter to you will understand and be there waiting to re-connect with you when you come up for air. Don't waste any energy on guilt.

10. The only person who will get you over the line is you, so be kind to yourself, park the negativity and believe in who you are. This is a skill that for most, takes training!

Whatever is given to us by the past, is adapted to the possibilities and demands of the future.

(Carl Jung, 1930)

For Your Support Team/Family/Friends 15

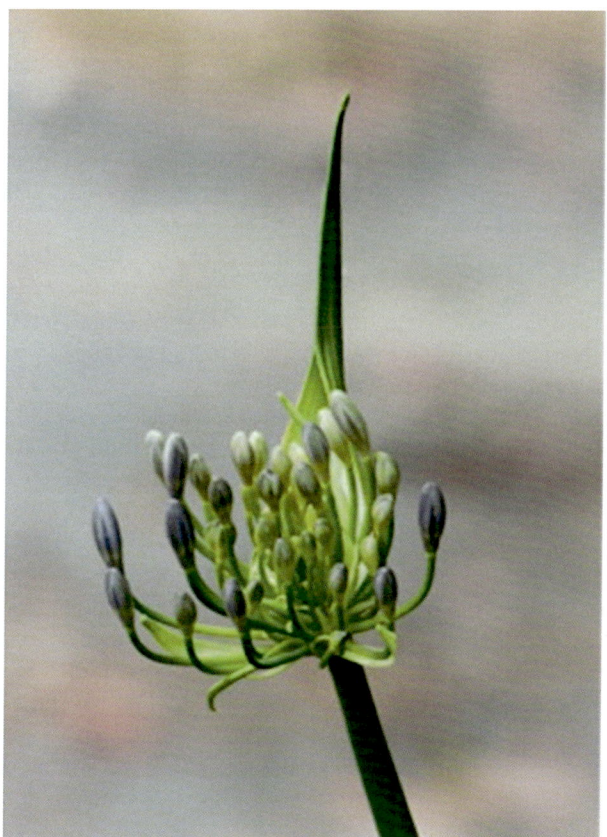

Agapanthus

Katerine Scott and Henry Willis contributed significantly to this chapter.

© Springer Nature Singapore Pte Ltd. 2018
M. F. Klaassen and E. Brown, *An Examiner's Guide to Professional
Plastic Surgery Exams*, https://doi.org/10.1007/978-981-13-0689-1_15

15.1   To the Families, Friends and Partners of Surgeons: "You're All in It Together"

We've spoken to some of the friends and family of surgeons who have repeated their exams and pulled together some top tips that it might be worth sharing with your loved ones at the outset so they too, know what to expect as you begin to sit—or resit the exam.

The biggest thing you need to come to grips with is accepting that while your 'student' has put their life on hold to get these exams done—yours is on hold too. This fact is even more pertinent when they don't pass the exam on the first run and the period of time goes from 'just 6 months in the grand scheme of things', to what feels like years on end—and the light at the end of the tunnel seems a lot further away. Here's a few tips from friends and families we spoke to that might help to remember along the way:

- *Don't underestimate the time needed to recover from failure*: The energy—emotional and physical—that has gone into sitting the exam is almost unfathomable to those outside the 'bubble' we are in. Recovering from a failure of any kind where you've put in this much effort isn't easy—but then throw into that the 'typical' personalities of surgical students and that is magnified. Your once unflappable and composed student will need time to recover—to work through it, to come to terms with his or her own fallibility and to be able to stomach starting it all over again. Don't underestimate how long this might take. Plan a holiday, lock the study door, and don't encourage them to get back to it too early. They need to be really ready to start again afresh, and this will take different amount of time for different people. Just let it take its course and be ready to restart your supporting role again with renewed enthusiasm too.
- *The support crew needs support too*: your role as chief cheerleader is relentless, often thankless and probably not one you've got much experience in. You too need an outlet for your frustrations, fears and pressure too. So make sure you have people you can unwind with and unload on, and can set aside time for you to take a break from the exams.
- *Always be ready with a set of 'mood boosters'*: the life of a supporter can be very up and down—depending on how the day of study has gone. Your student isn't just studying for this exam, they're holding down a very demanding job, dealing with the pressures of surgery, sometimes trying to be a parent too. But you know them best and they need you to intuitively know when they need a boost. Have a bank of things you can pull out to break the circuit, change the direction of a bad day, give them a break (that they won't feel guilty about taking). It could be as simple as their favourite treat food, a massage, a run or boxing session, something to brighten their study space … whatever suits them.
- *Remember who they were before this all started—they're possessed right now*: The person you knew is away for a while, but they WILL come back. This means that most things you demanded or expected of them are off the table. You have to lower and remove expectations around things like remembering birthdays,

returning phone calls, catching up for a spontaneous drink, replying to texts, turning up to family events, etc. For parents and partners this can be especially tough—but the last thing your student needs is to feel guilt or pressure from anything other than the exam. Passing it after having failed raises the stakes tenfold.

- *It's not about you*: This exam is the single biggest (career) thing your student will ever go through. In the main that means that whatever you have going on is—temporarily—of zero interest to them right now! But don't take it personally, they do really care, but just not right now. For partners going through their own family, work or friendship troubles this can be very isolating and you can mistake their lack of interest for something bigger than it is. Usually, it's just that it's not about you right now—it will be again, but not until they've passed and shaken the stigma of failure! Refer to the above point about having alternative support people for you.

- *Don't call them, they'll call you*: Every free moment for your student is probably being spent studying, thinking about studying or feeling guilty for not studying. So if they aren't studying then it's probably something else essential to life (eating, showering, sleeping!). Think about your contact with them—let them know you're there if they need, but leave them to contact you. There is nothing like a full inbox of unopened texts and emails from family and friends to make your student feel like they are losing control of their life. If you do get to spend precious time together, make it count!

- *At the end of the day, just get on with it:* Very wise words from a male partner of a surgical student! It's not your exam, but it is your life too. While some big things might be on hold you're the one who has to keep the wheels turning, the house functioning, the bills paid, the family on track. So your student just needs you to get on with it—and you need it for yourself too. When you're faced with their failures and disappointments they need sympathy and empathy, but they also need you to keep a stiff upper lip. You'll be disappointed too—but trust us—nothing you feel can eclipse their own internal feelings. Be pragmatic, let them know that you've got this and just get on with it.

Summary and General Advice

16

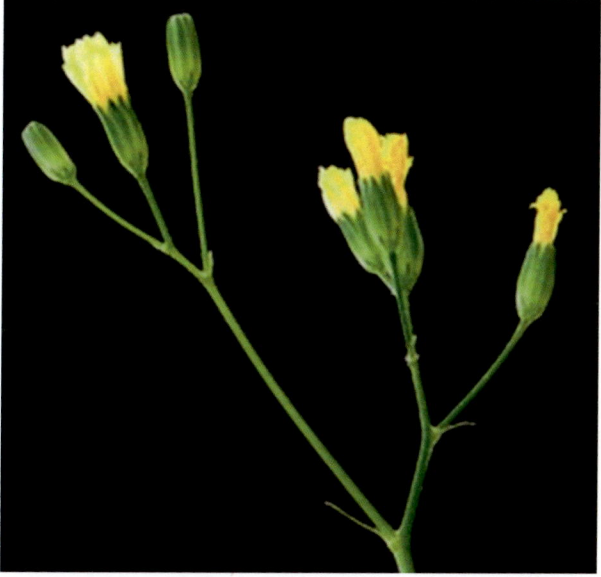

Lapsana Communis II

There is never a second opportunity to give a first impression
(Renato Saltz)

The well-prepared candidate should not fear professional plastic surgery exams.

The candidate who feels ready to present and has this confirmed by his/her supervisors/mentors should do so with quiet confidence.

© Springer Nature Singapore Pte Ltd. 2018
M. F. Klaassen and E. Brown, *An Examiner's Guide to Professional Plastic Surgery Exams*, https://doi.org/10.1007/978-981-13-0689-1_16

The candidate who doesn't feel confident but is encouraged by their supervisors/mentors needs to read this book and practice, practice, practice for the exam environment and interactions.

Communication is the key. Communicate your knowledge and experience to the examiner. Good communication skills carry you through your professional life, (hopefully keep you out of trouble) and make you a good Doctor.

Overconfidence and brashness can come across negatively and sew doubt into the examiners' minds.

All candidates must be healthy in mind and body to present their best face and performance. Professional Plastic Surgery Exams like the final FRACS, are the mental equivalent of running a marathon. Prepare your brain for a challenging test, that requires physical and mental toughness for success.

Saturation study and cramming just before the exams are due to commence, are always counter-productive to success.

Writing skills may not come naturally and require practice too. This skill can be refined in your clinic dictation notes.

Learn to construct precise, carefully worded prose that is meaningful and will catch the attention of an examiner, faced with many answers to mark. The good candidates stand out like beacons of light. At the beginning, define the exact point of the question and deconstruct this with an answer plan in bullet points, headlines or an algorithm of connected boxes/shapes.

Less is more in writing, and will ensure the reader is engaged. Keep your answers brief, interesting and don't be afraid to use your own style. Underline key words and concepts/principles. As Gillies once wrote, 'A good style in plastic surgery, will get you through'.

Start well and finish well. The intervening body of text should be in harmony with the beginning and the end.

Example: Ulcerated SCC left nasal vestibule (see Chap. 2).

START—'*The image illustrates an aggressive looking ulcerated tumour infiltrating the left columella, which has sinister implications for clinical severity and the need for a major resection and staged complex reconstruction of a key facial landmark*'.

BODY OF TEXT: 'Workup, imaging, biopsy, MDT, combined chemoradiation/ surgery, immediate versus delayed reconstruction, CLEAR versus DRAPE, anaesthetic considerations PACS (Proper Anaesthetic Care & Safety), different stages of reconstruction, anticipated potential complications, prognosis, survival chances, consideration of prosthetic versus autologous reconstruction'.

FINISH—'*Non-healing ulcerative lesions involving the aerodigestive tract of chronic smokers should raise the possibility of malignancy early. The earlier these lesions are diagnosed the more successful the potential outcomes. Never underestimate the challenge for the patient and family of disfiguring ablative surgery and complex staged reconstruction in terms of time, energy and mental well-being*'.

The good candidate will always consider plastic surgery principles, alternative management options, risks and complications and most importantly the patient's feelings and feedback.

Fig. 16.1 The case from chapter 2 of an ulcerated lesion involving the columellar and caudal septum in a chronic smoker

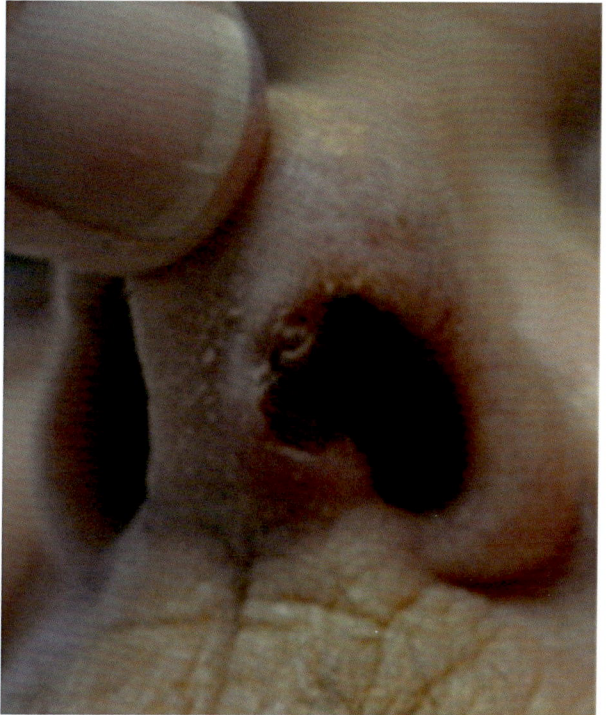

There is some value in quoting pioneers of a particular branch of plastic surgery. For the nasal cancer case above (Fig. 16.1), the treatment plan was based on the important principles of aesthetic nasal reconstruction as defined by the late Gary Burget and Fred Menick. These Principles were earlier promoted by Ralph Millard based on the Sir Harold Gillies Commandments (Chap. 4) (based on what had been passed down to them via Ralph Millard Jnr and to him by Sir Harold Gillies CBE). It is probably not helpful though to excessively quote the recent medical literature where some novel idea or concept may not yet be broadly tested or accepted by everyone. An appreciation of the historical evolution of techniques and surgical methods, however, shows a maturity of understanding and reflection.

Oral skills of communication are mandatory for a large part of the professional plastic surgery exams. Some candidates are natural orators, confident and good at thinking and articulating on their feet.

Others will have to spend time practising this so that during the exam process, it may come naturally too. There are some basic principles to be remembered here:

Stay calm and friendly, smile occasionally to disarm your examiners.

Make eye contact from time to time.

Show compassion and consideration for the patient you are examining.

Learn to speak slowly with clear articulation and give the impression that you are thinking and speaking like a new surgeon consultant. It can be a challenge to break away from the role model of a trainee, but this is important for overall exam success.

In the marking of hundreds of mock/practice exam answers over the past 5 years my most common feedback was:

> Start thinking and writing like a consultant plastic surgeon, rather than a time-expired trainee. Take ownership and responsibility for the clinical problem before you and based on sound and ageless fundamental principles, make good clinical decisions based on the evidence, the signs and the circumstances for the patient & problem.

A suggested template for this is:

1. What is the problem?
2. Is it simple or complex?
3. Are there extenuating circumstances, patient risk factors, atypical features?
4. Is there tissue missing or displaced? (W M Machester)
5. Diagnose before you treat (H D Gillies)
6. Don't let routine method become your master (H D Gillies)
7. Make a plan and a pattern (H D Gillies)
8. Do something positive (H D Gillies)
9. What could I do here?
10. What do I favour as a method?
11. What should I do after considering 9 & 10.
12. Always have a backup plan and a lifeboat (H D Gillies)
13. Don't be too proud or arrogant to 'cry for help'—consult other specialists (H D Gillies)

Some other variables to consider for every clinical case:

1. Co-morbidities involving the cardiovascular system, lungs, kidneys and liver.
2. Extrinsic factors such as drugs, tobacco and alcohol.
3. Intrinsic factors such as degenerative diseases, immunosuppression, diabetes mellitus, hypertension, anticoagulation, nutrition, cognitive dysfunction (dementia, depression and body dysmorphic syndrome).

Complex discussions with the patient should be managed in supportive, open-minded conversations, about what they understand about the diagnosis, the options for management and their personal wishes.

Complex congenital anomalies should always be managed in an MDT setting, with protocol-based treatment programmes applied with sound strategies over a time scale, from childhood—teenage years—adult years.

Aesthetic problems should always be considered in the context of applied anatomy, the physiology of aging and the breadth of treatment methods from simple to extended. The driving agenda and motivations of the patient contrasted with their personality profile are also essential considerations.

Appendix A: Model Answers to Written Questions (Chap. 5)

Mock 01

Plan A 32-yr-old female incomplete left breast reconstruction/declines further stages/images to discuss/her decision is significant and warrants consideration/what is the risk of recurrent breast cancer/what are her plans for life/what support does she have at home and from extended family/what do young women with breast cancer prioritise in terms of form, function, survival? Should adjuvant chemo-radiation be considered in the management plan?

Answer The images show a young woman of normal BMI post total left mastectomy. Breast drawings indicate plans for staged reconstruction. The contralateral (right) breast has an aesthetic form with some ptosis. She does not look like she would be a candidate for a TRAM flap or variant due to lack of donor tissue. The second and third images show a completed left breast reconstruction with absence of the NAC and some asymmetry with the contralateral breast, but I would assume that she looks reasonably symmetrical in clothing, including swimwear (she is a marine biologist). Her decision to decline further refinements and reconstruction is entirely reasonable and I would accept this and encourage her to move on with her life and career, but happy to re-consider her reconstructive needs anytime in the future. I would liaise closely with her breast oncological surgeon and other oncological team members. Her pathology is significant (extensive DCIS with foci of invasion) and clearly there are surveillance and follow-up issues going forward. What is the true risk of breast cancer recurrence for this patient? Could this be at her left mastectomy site and scar, locally? Ideally her left mastectomy scar should have sent for histology at the first stage of her staged left breast reconstruction with Latissimus Dorsi flap + Tissue expander followed by definitive Implant. Regional recurrence in her left axilla or an asychronous new breast cancer in her remaining right breast are also oncological considerations. She is nulliparous age 32 years, so the risk of further breast cancer may still be significant. Should she have the genetic BRCA gene tests? Although a right mastopexy would be straight-forward this is an aesthetic

© Springer Nature Singapore Pte Ltd. 2018
M. F. Klaassen and E. Brown, *An Examiner's Guide to Professional Plastic Surgery Exams*, https://doi.org/10.1007/978-981-13-0689-1

issue and if she is comfortable and confident with her current appearance then that is the PRIORITY. I have heard clinical psychologists associated with Breast Cancer Care teams discuss the priorities of different patients, at different stages of their lives and careers. For most young women with breast cancer the risk of the breast cancer returning is their Big worry. How long will the disease-free interval be, will they develop stage 2, 3 or 4 breast cancer at some stage in the future? Will a patient like this 32-year-old scientist and otherwise healthy woman, wish to have children? Will she be around to see them grow and develop to become teenagers and then adults? These family and survival issues are probably much more pressing than a perfectly symmetrical breast reconstruction, with a reconstructed NAC and a perfectly aligned inframammary fold. This question implies to me the importance of connectedness with your patient, so clearly defined by Sir Archibald McIndoe. We must listen to what they want, and support their decisions. Her decision to decline further reconstruction at this stage is reasonable, practicable and one her surgeon should respect.

Mock 02

Plan Skin cancer of different regions of the face/cutaneous defects needing repair/is there tissue missing or displaced?/will direct repair be possible or will new tissue have to be imported/an algorithm or tabular form of answer seems reasonable here. In the general plan for repair, always consider where there are areas of 'spare' skin.

Answer

Face region	Types of skin cancer	Preferred method of repair
Scalp	SCC, BCC, melanoma, sarcoma	Split skin or FTSG in the elderly
		Rotation local flaps +/− SSG to donor
		Keystone local flaps can work but need experience
Forehead	SCC, BCC, melanoma	Direct closure may be possible, especially in the glabellar region
		Biwinged method avoids landmark distortion (eyebrow, hairline)
		H-plasty for smaller defects
		Total forehead rotation/advancement flap for larger defects
		Small defects and even moderate defects will heal well by auto-contraction
Upper eyelid region	BCC, SCC, rarely sebaceous CA	Direct closure as for blepharoplasty and direct closure of full thickness eyelid defect for up to 1/4 of the lid
		Full thickness skin graft from contralateral upper eyelid
		Mustardé lower lid switch flap + formal reconstruction of lower lid with * (subtotal loss)

(continued)

Face region	Types of skin cancer	Preferred method of repair
Lower eyelid	BCC, SCC, rarely sebaceous CA	Wedge resection +/− lateral canthotomy for defects up to 1/3 of the lower lid
		Mustardé or *McGregor rotation flaps +/− lateral canthotomy +/− chondromucosal or palatal mucosal graft for conjunctival lining for vertical defects
		Tripier unipedicle or bipedicle upper lid flaps for horizontal defects +/− chondromucosal or palatal mucosal grafts
Temporal region	BCC, SCC, melanoma	Direct closure, rotation flaps, keystone flaps
Zygomatic/ preauricular	BCC, SCC, melanoma	Direct closure, keystone flap, facelift flap
		Postauricular interpolated flap with SSG to secondary defect
		Modified rhomboid transposition flap
Mid cheek/ medial	BCC, SCC, melanoma	Ono's sigmoid oblique advancement flap
		Cervico-facial rotation flaps
Medial canthus	BCC	Banner transposition flap
		Glabellar transposition flap
		Full thickness skin graft (pre or postauricular)
Nose	BCC, SCC, SCC in-situ	Direct closure if possible on dorsum, side-wall
		Aesthetic subunit full thickness grafts in the elderly
		2-stage nasolabial interpolated flap + cartilage graft for alar subunit in the young and elderly
		Nasoaxial V-Y advancement flaps for supratip and tip (can utilise cosmetic rhinoplasty principles of tip reduction)
		Paramedian forehead flap for tip, dorsum and subtotal or total defects. Needs at least three stages
Ear	BCC, SCC, melanoma, CDNH	Composite wedge + rotation advancement
		Postauricular interpolated flaps for anterior ear
		Mastoid flap or preauricular interpolated flap for conchal defects
		Temporalis fascial flap, cartilage framework and skin grafts for large subtotal ear defects
Upper lip	BCC, SCC, SCC in-situ	Direct closure in the relaxed skin tension lines (RSTLs)
		Asymmetrical sliding flap after wedge resection
		Perialar crescentic advancement flaps for central upper lip
Lower lip	SCC, dysplastic cheilitise, melanoma	Wedge resection
		Lip shave and mucosal advancement
		Keystone flaps
		Karapandzic neurovascular rotation flaps
		Bernard flaps with Burow's triangles
Chin	BCC, SCC	Direct closure in RSTLs
		Various keystone flap designs
Neck	BCC, SCC, melanoma	Often direct closure utilising lax neck skin

Local flaps are favoured and repair of the aesthetic subunit as a principle, when >50% of the unit is lost with the cancer excision.

The elderly tolerate full thickness skin grafts very well though colour mismatch can be a problem.

Convex surfaces like the nasal tip and nasal alar are better repaired with flaps and sometimes structural support is required under the flap utilising cartilage grafts from either the concha or septum.

In staged local flap repairs don't over-thin the flap at second stage and be prepared to return in 6 months for final contouring.

In young patients where scar disfigurement is a concern, healing by secondary intention may give an excellent aesthetic result with the smallest overall scar.

Mock 03

Plan The spectrum of hand fractures: simple vs complex, low velocity vs high velocity, stable vs unstable, intra-articular vs extra-articular, compound vs closed, multiple vs single fractures, small versus large soft tissue defects, special fractures, patient factors, timing of surgery, aftercare/splintage, hand therapy and rehabilitation, complex regional pain syndromes. Optimal use of radiology imaging modalities is also important in the overall consideration.

Answer The spectrum of hand fractures is diverse, from crushed nail bed fingertip injuries in children to low velocity phalangeal/metacarpal fractures in sport, to high velocity complex injuries in road and industrial trauma, to catastrophic injuries from gunshot wounds and other explosive devices. The mechanism of injury will determine the severity of damage and the management plan. Patient factors such as hand dominance, occupation, musicianship, sports involvement, general health, motivation and reliability are all key factors. Diagnose before you treat: history, examination and imaging (X-ray, CT or MRI). Informed consent. Anaesthetic considerations—regional versus general anaesthetic. Salvage of the damaged digit versus sacrifice. Terminalisation versus ray amputation. Associated soft tissue, tendon and nerve damage. Crush injuries are the most devitalising and potentially the most challenging long-term with chronic pain and dysfunction. Have a plan and a pattern. Have a lifeboat. Emergency versus delayed primary repair, particularly if post-trauma swelling needs to resolve. A good principle is to stabilise hand fractures before soft tissue repair. The most severe fracture is an amputation, where replantation should be considered. The key emphasis is the RESTORATION of hand FUNCTION. Safe hand immobilisation in the COBRA position (wrist extended, MCPJs flexed 90°, PIPJs extended) to maintain ligamentous stretch, elevation (Bradford arm slings or similar). Temporary stabilisation of unstable fractures in a volar slab, buddy tapping of with Kirschner wires. Perioperative surgery, tourniquet safety, antibiotic prophylaxis and other strategies to prevent surgical site infection. Unstable intra-articular fractures require open reduction and internal fixation with either K-wires or mini-plates and screws. External fixation with K-wire scaffolds also possible. ORIF allows for primary wound closure and early hand mobilisation. Contaminated joint fractures, soft tissue loss and tendon or nerve damage may require more complex reconstructions with nerve grafts, tendon grafts, bone grafts and flap cover. Decisions about the long-term viability and function of a digit may be conversations to be held once the true prognosis is revealed. In general principle keep the surgery as simple as possible, to facilitate primary bone healing whilst maintaining hand movements and function. Specialist hand therapists should be part of the rehabilitation team from day one. Post-operative pain in certain crushing or mangling injuries may need anaesthetic/pain team management. Specialised injures: Volar plate ruptures, pelon fractures of the PIPJ, spiral fractures of the metacarpals with angulation and scissor deformity, Bennett's fracture/dislocation of the base of the first metacarpal, scaphoid fractures with non-union, wrist fractures including Colles fracture, Smith's fracture, distal radio-ulnar joint disruption, pathological fractures through bone cysts. Immobilisation of the hand after age 45 is poorly tolerated and stiffness may be a significant problem. Remember that a patient is attached to the hand and it is as important to treat the patient as their specific hand fracture—this requires compassion, experience and professionalism. Occupational therapists and even occupation medicine specialists have important roles. Third parties like ACC, insurance companies and employers are also part of the equation. There are often medico-legal implications and issues. The ultimate success or failure of any hand fracture hangs in a multifactorial balance, where patient factors, surgeon factors and environment factors all play a role.

Mock 04

Plan Priority is the BCC infiltrating the woman's right conchal fossa, wide excision and immediate reconstruction to prevent local recurrence. Can this be combined with a mini-facelift? Complete excision of the BCC is paramount. What sources of skin are available for the repair? Should combined or separate procedures be selected?

Answer The first image shows an ulcerated infiltrating BCC located in the right concha with planned excision margins likely to involve all the skin and underlying cartilage of the cavum concha. My usual method of choice for these defects is the mastoid island local flap, sometimes known as the 'revolving door flap'. The mastoid island flap is planned opposite the proposed surgical defect, in the postauricular sulcus. It is islanded so that it will advance 90 degrees to restore skin to the defect. Alternative options include: free skin grafts (full thickness or split thickness) and loco-regional flaps that can be interpolated into the defect from areas of relative laxity. The image also shows some preauricular skin laxity and her AP face view shows the early signs of cheek and jawline laxity associated with atrophy and ageing in middle-age. An inferiorly based preauricular flap of 15 mm width could be raised to the level of the earlobe and tunnelled under the earlobe into the conchal defect. The bridging part would need to be carefully de-epithelialised to avoid devascularising the local flap. The right preauricular donor defect would then need closing and this could be achieved with the anterior flicklift mini-facelift described by Frame and Levick from England in 2002. This involves a triangular SMAS flap that is lifted cephalad and fixed to the deep temporal fascia with a strong figure of 8 suture and the preauricular defect is repaired by the advancing lateral cheek skin. It would be necessary to perform a similar anterior flicklift on the contralateral side and this could be timed to be done synchronously or at some later date. The combination of a preauricular local flap interpolated to make good the cutaneous/cartilaginous right conchal defect with a minifacelift is one method appropriate for this patient's needs and wishes. Anaesthesia options: local anaesthetic alone or combined with intravenous sedation as a day case.

Mock 05

Plan Rhinoplasty—reconstructive vs aesthetic, functional vs form, open vs closed, associated techniques—airway, septoplasty, turbinate reduction, endoscopic sinus surgery. COMPARE & CONTRAST/multidisciplinary/psychological/informed consent/complications.

Answer A consideration of the techniques of rhinoplasty is a journey through the historic evolution of plastic surgery itself. From the earliest attempts at nose repair by the ancient caste of Indian potters circa 600 BC, the inner arm pedicle flaps of Tagliacozzi (sixteenth century Bologne), Gillies forehead flaps with bovine cartilage (circa 1914–1918) and the modern principles of aesthetic nose reconstruction so well defined by Burget and Menick in the 1990s. Rhinoplasty per se is the surgery to correct the shape and function of the nose. A full rhinoplasty may involve a hump removal, osteotomies (medial and lateral), infracturing to reduce the open roof and size of the bony vault, cartilage modifications and tip refinement. The lateral profile of the face should always be considered in the aesthetic assessment for rhinoplasty because sometimes an 'ugly' nose can be exaggerated by a small chin. Chin augmentation with implant or sliding genioplasty may be required. The dental occlusion should also be assessed because maxillary orthognathic problems as well as mandibular problems may be contributing. More conservative rhinoplasty surgery may involve just tip refinement to correct a drooping tip of, for instance, an Arabic nose, or the bulbous poorly defined tip of a Polynesian nose. The cleft lip nasal deformity is a very specific challenge associated with hypoplasia of the underlying hemi-maxilla as well as slumping and displacement of the lateral lower cartilage crus. The deviated nose either from acquired trauma or congenital deviation from traumatic childbirth has its own challenges to reconstruct deviated cartilage and bony structures to correct airway obstruction. Rhinophyma is a particular entity, the severest form of rosacea which cripples the patient with a disfiguring large and bulbous nose, which is simply resected using tangential shave method under general anaesthetic. Traditional rhinoplasty techniques and instrumentation were developed and pioneered by Jacques Joseph of Berlin and his results in the 1931 publication

Rhinoplastik, are truly impressive. Students of Joseph like Aufricht who moved from Berlin to New York during the second world war lead to further improvements in understanding and application of the techniques of rhinoplasty. Sheen, Millard, Burget and others have continued this evolution. The closed approach is my favoured but is also the most difficult technically. The open approach is the easiest to perform and from which to learn the skill-set required for competent rhinoplasty but it is more invasive, creates more scarring and significantly more tip swelling in the post-operative weeks. The closed approach requires magnification and a good headlight. Incisions are planned endonasally via the intercartilaginous or intracartilaginous route with transfixion incision connecting via the caudal end of the septum. Osteotomy access is either via the nasal vestibules, the buccal sulcus (guarded oste-otomies) or externally through the sidewall skin with mini osteotomies. Septal mucosal dissection is critical and the anatomical plane between cartilage and adherent nasal mucosa important to enter atraumatically. Cartilage deviation and distortion is best corrected with either septoplasty or septal resection techniques. Turbinectomy or turbinate outfracturing are alternative options for difficult airways. The open approach is performed through a columellar stair-step incision at the nar-row segment of the columellar and connecting to vestibular incisions which are continued cephalad inside the nostril rims. Careful dissection over the domes of the tip cartilages then allows the dorsal/tip/columellar skin flap to be lifted and all the cartilage structures are revealed. Special retractors delicately retract the soft tissues without causing ischaemic damage. The open approach just described gives the surgeon excellent exposure of the anatomical variation in form of the lower lateral cartilages, much clearer than even the delivery techniques of the closed approach. After trimming, cartilage suturing or even adding cartilage grafts to the tip structure, the skin is re-draped and the stair-step incision closed with fine sutures. Absorbable sutures (catgut) are used to repair the mucosal wounds. Intra-nasal packing with foam packing splints and external splinatge should be considered to complete the repair. For secondary or tertiary rhinoplasty, I find the open approach almost manda-tory but for the standard conservative primary rhinoplasty the closed approach is simpler, faster and very convenient. Each rhinoplasty case is unique and a varied range of surgical approaches and surgical techniques is available—e.g. short nose, long nose, bulbous nose, saddle nose, ethnic nose, bifid nose, etc.

Mock 06

Plan Neonatal ear moulding: theory & practice/cartilage maturation with growth/ hormones of pregnancy/deformations/anatomy/techniques/historical developments/ success/complications.

Answer The Japanese plastic surgeons were the first to popularise the moulding of neonatal ear deformities in the 1980s with the use of simple materials available from any DIY or hardware store. Gault and Tan refined this in the UK and commer-cialised the EarBuddie™, followed soon after by the Earwell™, which is a USA device. The ears of newborn babies and toddlers are very soft and malleable, so that any deformities they may have, are very suitable for treatment by moulding. As the child grows their auricular cartilage becomes firmer and will conform to the new shape influenced by the moulding process. The earlier the moulding is commenced the less time it takes to achieve the ideal aesthetic shape. Starting early, say in the first 2 weeks of life necessitates only between 2 and 3 weeks of active moulding. From 3 to 5 months of age the moulding may need to continue for 3–4 months. I have successfully moulded the prominent upper poles of a 11-month-old child, which took 4 months. Eventually some parents will become confident enough to apply and remove the moulds themselves. Some training and encouragement from the practitioner is needed. The deformities correctable by ear moulding include: prominent ears, lop ears, constricted ears, Stahl's ear, chicane ear, prominent ear lobes, kinks of the helical rim, cryptotia and kinks in the antihelical fold. Malformations with missing tissue such as microtia and its variants are unsuitable. The best and easily available moulding material is lead-free soldering wire, covered with Fixomull tape. Make sure there are no sharp ends and fix the shaped splint to the ear, inside the helical rim with Micropore tape or Steristrips. The moulding process is completed by overcorrection, with taping the ear back to the previously shaved temporal and postauricular scalp. I recommend changing the splints every 2 weeks and checking for skin irritation and potential dislodgement of the splints. The results in my hands over 5 years have been impressive and the only failures have been when the parents decided to abandon the method. Complications have been few and the most common in about 10% of children is contact dermatitis from the adhesive backing of the Fixomull tape. The answer is to switch to broader Micropore tape which is hypoallergenic. I believe the aesthetic results from ear moulding produce much more natural looking, scar less ear forms, than any of the otoplasty techniques I have used. Otoplasty after the age of 8–9 years is the backup plan.

Mock 07

Plan A 20-yr-old female suffering from Ehlers-Danlos syndrome requests bilateral breast reduction. Risks of the surgery, added risks of the syndrome/anaesthetic/surgical/co-morbidities/surgical implications/Management strategies should consider preoperative workup/intraoperative strategies/post-operative care/informed consent/teamwork. Briefly describe the syndrome named after Ehlers-Danlos and this patient's past history of EDS problems.

Answer Ehlers-Danlos syndrome is a rare but serious condition with generalised disorder of the connective tissues affecting multiple organs. The history suggests that this is not a typical breast reduction case. Chronic pain management for joint instabilities—which joints? Could be cervical spine, thoracic spine, major limb joints such as gleno-humeral instability. Thoracic outlet syndrome with two previous first rib resections. The outcome and anaesthetic issues related to these episodes should be documented somewhere and needs review. I would ask her consultant rheumatologist for a briefing from a medical perspective and also ask an experienced anaesthetist to review her from the perianaesthetic risk perspective. Do these patients have cardiac abnormalities or any other significant risk factors such as cardiovascular instability and/or bleeding tendencies? Cardiology workup may also be indicated.

Attention then turns to the breast hypertrophy problem itself. The image shows severe ptosis for a young woman, nulliparous and this has probably both functional and aesthetic concerns for her, including chest wall compliance and symptoms from the biomechanical load. Her motivations, understanding and expectations all need to be discussed in supportive, compassionate conversations. From the image (Fig. 5.3) her Suprasternal notch-nipple distances are 31–30 cm and her Inframammary Fold (horizontal reference plane for new NAC position) level is marked as 22 cm, so, this is a significant lift of the NAC. The distance the NAC will be lifted on the dermoglandular pedicle is $31 - 22 = 9.0$ cm. All the usual potential problems of breast reduction surgery need to be considered along with the added risks contributed to by her condition. A hospital with intensive care facilities should be selected and collaboration needs to occur between all the medical, anaesthetic and surgical teams. The specific surgical concerns would include wound healing, suture stability and bleeding problems. I would plan to use non-absorbable sutures for internal suturing and surgical drains for each breast. I would be advising her that we should have as a goal a B cup breast size. The peri-operative plan would be worked out in collaboration with the consultant anaesthetist and the theatre nursing team, as well as recovery team and ward nurses. Positioning, monitoring, splinting of cervical spine and plasma products on induction would all be considered. I would advise her to be an inpatient for at least 2–4 days depending on her progress. I would search the literature to try and find if there was any general experience with surgery for patients with EDS. There is of course the potential greater risk of post operative ptosis due to the EDS. I would consult trusted colleagues for the same. Finally, a careful informed consent would be constructed and further discussions leading up to the surgery with patient and her family. The priorities would always be safety and minimisation of complications.

Mock 08

Plan Athletic middle-aged physique with breast involution/hypoplasia associated with ptosis. Volume and lift both desired but without breast implants. Options, risks and expectations. The conversation and the justification for recommendations.

Answer This is a difficult case because of the grade 3 bilateral breast ptosis (Fig. 5.4) on a fit woman of normal BMI and body habitus. The image does not show much spare abdominal fat for fat grafts and there seems to be an associated periumbilical hernia. The patient looks as though she works out in a gym and has well-developed pectoralis major muscles. There are also some skin lesions marked, presumably moles or papillomata. Her SSN-N distance is marked as 23–24 cm and the IMF level or horizontal plane, measured from the SSN is marked as 20 cm. This makes a vertical mastopexy, straightforward, using the modified technique of Dr. Madeleine Lejour. The volume deficit will be a problem even after re-positioning of the breast parenchyma with plication and folding. I would recommend that before the breast lift proper, I would harvest as much fat as possible from her abdomen, thighs and lateral buttocks and use this according to the Liposculpture technique of Dr. Sydney Coleman, to augment the breast volume. For a novice surgeon, a safe plan may be to start with the fat grafting and then perform mastopexy at a second stage. Alternatively, the surgeon could perform a bilateral mastopexy and later add fat grafting to the breast volume at a second stage. These options mean two procedures and two anaesthetics with the added costs for the patient. I would therefore recommend one stage fat graft breast augmentation combined simultaneously with Lejour style mastopexy. Further fat grafting +/− breast implants could be considered if the desired result is not met for the patient. If she still resists breast implants (which is understandable and reasonable), then serial fat grafting could be a maintenance option going forward until the desired breast form, shape and projection is achieved. The usual warnings about potential risks, hazards and complications for both breast surgery and fat grafting would be discussed including: asymmetry, infection, haematoma, seroma, fat necrosis, scars, dysasethesia, numbness, loss of erogenous sensation and need for further surgery. The discussion would need to be specific and make sure the patient's expectations are understood. A PowerPoint presentation with illustration of other similar breast problem cases would be beneficial for helping the patient make an informed choice. The volume of fat available for grafting would be the critical factor and ideally, I would be hoping to add 80– 100 cc of fat grafts to each breast. This is a case where connectedness with the patient and surgical experience are extremely important to the outcome.

Appendix B: Ralph Millard's Expanded Gillies' Principles

Preparational Principles

1. Priorities

    'Correct the order of priorities'. Applied broadly, this could mean emphasizing integrity and ethics; it could mean prioritizing function over form; and it could also mean performing a blepharoplasty before a facelift since the latter could affect the former but not vice versa. The bottom line is that whether in life or in a specific procedure, each part needs to be considered in the context of the whole.

2. Aptitude

    'Aptitude should determine specialization', meaning that the plastic surgeon should play to strengths when deciding whether to focus on reconstructive surgery, cosmetic surgery, microvascular surgery, craniofacial surgery, head and neck oncology, hand surgery, burn physiology or laboratory research.

3. Second abilities

    'Mobilize auxiliary capabilities'. That is to say, the plastic surgeon should incorporate individual talents to develop a 'personal style with individual flair'. Advised to develop one primary capability and several secondary talents such as sculpture, music, writing or painting, the ideal plastic surgeon would be multi-talented for maximal depth and versatility in the operating room.

4. No harm

    'Acknowledge your limitations so as to do no harm', a self-evident principle that speaks to the temptation to persevere on a case with endless complications. Instead, the successful surgeon should know when to stop.

5. Most good

    'Extend your abilities to do the most good'. This speaks to the moral obligation to use plastic surgical training to alleviate human suffering, that is, to reconstruct mutilated or severely deformed patients instead of limiting one's practice to purely aesthetic procedures.

6. Patient's desires

    'Seek insight into the patient's true desires'. Delving into the psyche, this principle directs the plastic surgeon to decipher a patient's actual problems instead of merely taking the stated problem at face value to pre-empt patient disappointment, improve public relations and prevent postoperative legal complications. Communication.

7. Goal
   'Have a goal and a dream'. In plastic surgery, this principle shifts depending on whether a procedure is primarily cosmetic, in which the goal would be to surpass normal, or primarily reconstructive, in which the goal would be to attain normal. Either way, the plastic surgeon should have a target in mind before beginning an operation.

8. Beautiful normal
   'Know the ideal beautiful normal'. While this ideal beautiful normal can vary among different ethnic backgrounds, it was important for the plastic surgeon to be able to define it in order to attain pleasing aesthetic proportions and visual harmony.

9. Literature
   'Be familiar with the literature'. Knowing what has already been described assists a surgeon in discriminating between procedures that would and would not be successful; it also gives the surgeon access to a collective bank of experience that allows extension beyond what one person could accrue in a lifetime.

10. Record
    'Keep an accurate record' was like the sixth principle in that its underlying purpose was both to further patient care and provide legal protection for the surgeon. In addition, since memory is inherently unreliable, accurate written and photographic records provided baseline references that allow the plastic surgeon to coordinate multi-staged procedures to achieve a successful final result. Communication.

11. Condition/position
    'Attend to physical condition and comfort of position'. Often overlooked by single-minded surgeons, the basis of this principle was the belief that the optimal surgical performance depended upon good physical condition and a comfortable working position for the surgeon.

12. Know foe
    'Do not underestimate the enemy' acknowledges that peril lies behind every procedure. Thus, whether the enemy is hypertrophic scar formation or inadequate vascular supply, it is never possible to be overly vigilant in preventing surgical complications

Executional Principles

13. Diagnose
    'Diagnose before treating' emphasized that observation was the basis of surgical diagnosis. The plastic surgeon must use all senses—particularly visual and tactile cues—to accurately determine a problem before proceeding with an operation.

14. Norm to norm

    This principle is reminiscent of Paré, in that it advised the plastic surgeon to 'return what is normal to normal position and retain it there'. As previously mentioned, displacement of structures could be due to failure in normal embryonic development or as a direct result of trauma, ablation, scar contraction, or even the aging process, but correction required the ability to recognize the norm in order to restore displaced parts to their correct place.

15. Like tissue

    'Tissue losses should be replaced in kind'. More specifically, when attempting reconstruction of lost body parts, bone should be replaced with bone, muscle with muscle and glabrous skin with glabrous skin. If exact replacement is impossible, then a similar substitute should be made, such as a beard with scalp, thin skin for an eyelid, thick skin for the sole of a foot, and a prosthesis for an eye. The idea is that replacing like with like would give the most natural outcome.

16. Units

    'Reconstruct by units'. By basing reconstruction on unit borders demarcated by creases, margins, angles and hairlines, surgical scars can often be concealed by the meeting of light and shadow.

17. Plan

    'Make a plan, a pattern and a second plan (lifeboat)'. By visualizing an entire operation from beginning to end, the plastic surgeon can anticipate possible difficulties and then proceed to devise a secondary plan for use should the primary plan fail.

18. Thrift

    'Invoke a Scot's economy'. This involves thrift in surgery, in which no tissue is ever discarded until it was certain that it was no longer needed. A corollary of this was to discard the useless, as once a piece of tissue was determined to have no further value it should be removed—but refrigerated storage was advised even then in case the tissue could be used later.

19. Robin Hood

    Robin Hood would steal from the rich to give to the poor. Likewise, this principle advises using excess tissue to make up for areas with tissue deficits by rotating, transposing, or transplanting expendable tissue flaps to areas in need.

20. Donor area

    'Consider the secondary donor site'. That is, while reconstructing deficient areas with tissue taken from areas that were more ample, the resulting secondary defect must also be considered to make sure that its sacrifice was not too deforming.

21. Tension

    'Learn to control tension'. In opening, tension usually facilitates a clean cut with the scalpel; in closure, tension could lead to tissue necrosis or excess scarring; in flap design, skin tension lines could be identified and used to camouflage scars.

22. Craft
    'Perfect your craftsmanship'. For the plastic surgeon, "good" suggests mediocrity, and nothing short of perfection is acceptable.
23. Caution
    'When in doubt, don't!' Doubt should function as a deterrent, and if a solution to a problem leaves seeds of doubt, it is better to develop a better idea.

Innovational Principles

24. Follow-up
    'Follow up with a critical eye'. That is, it is important to follow patients post-operatively over time to critically evaluate results, as regular review of one's handiwork is the best way to spur advancement and improvement of surgical procedures.
25. Flexibility
    'Avoid the rut of routine', exhorted surgeons to shun mindless and tenacious clinging to unthinking rituals. Again, by thinking outside the box, the plastic surgeon could make the advance to the next level of innovation and development.
26. Innovate
    'Imagination sparks innovation' is the 'breakthrough' or problem-solving principle that encourages free-spirited thinking and creativity.
27. Recovery
    'Think while down and turn a setback into a victory' is labelled the 'prince of principles' by Millard. It admonished the surgeon not to panic or despair, or compound error when faced with possible defeat. Instead, the surgeon should keep cool while determining the cause of loss, expend no energy in worrying about a compromised position, and make certain not to repeat the same mistake while thinking one's way to recovery.
28. Research
    'Research basic truths by laboratory experimentation'. By testing even minor theories in the laboratory, the surgeon could discover answers to plastic surgical questions in a controlled setting.

Contributional Principles

29. Other specialties
    'Gain access to other specialties' problems'. By consulting with physicians or surgeons from other specialties, it could be possible to learn management of common complications that would both benefit patients and broaden the base of plastic surgery.

30. Teaching

    'Teaching our specialty is its best legacy'. The implication was that the best way to extend plastic surgery was to transmit knowledge via lectures, books, symposiums and personal experiences to ensuing generations.

31. Missions

    'Participate in reconstructive missions'. Moreover, the ideal method to conduct such missions is to lend specialists not just to operate, but to teach people in underdeveloped countries how to perform the operations and manage all the postoperative care themselves.

Inspirational Principles

32. Go for broke

    'Go for broke!' That is, the plastic surgeon should use every means possible to overcome obstacles, strive for the very best, and seek perfection.

33. Automatic in m.o. modus operandi

    'Think principles until they become instinctively automatic in your modus operandi'. By incorporating principles constantly and consistently into plastic surgical practice, it would become second nature to avoid rote memorization of techniques and instead stimulate the imagination to engage in innovative problem solving.

    Ref: **Principalization** of Plastic Surgery D Ralph Millard 1986

The Plastic Surgeon's Creed

Condensing the 33 principles.

Know the ideal beautiful normal
Diagnose what is *present*, what is *diseased, destroyed, displaced, or distorted*, and what is in *excess*.
Then, guided by the normal in your mind's eye, utilise what you have to make what you *want*—and when possible *go for even better* than what would have been.

Appendix C: Recommended Reading List

Recommended Reading List

Gillies HD. Plastic surgery of the face – based on selected cases of war injuries of the face including burns. Facsimile Edition published by Gower Medical (1983); 1920.

Acland RD. Acland's DVD atlas of human anatomy. Vols. 1–5. Lippincott Williams and Wilkins; 2004

Klaassen MF, Brown E, Behan FC. Simply local flaps. Cham: Springer; 2018.

Richards AM. Key notes on plastic surgery. Great Britain: Blackwell Science; 2002.

Stone C. Plastic surgery facts. Greenwich Medical Media; 2001.

Olivari N. Practical plastic and reconstructive surgery: an atlas of operations and techniques. Heidelberg: Kaden; 2008.

Galler D. Things that matter: stories of life & death. Auckland: Allen and Unwin; 2016.

Banks P, Brown A. Fractures of the facial skeleton. Elsevier Science; 2002.

Lister G. The hand: diagnosis and indications. Churchill Livingstone; 1984.

Tubiana R, et al. Examination of the hand and wrist. Martin Dunitz; 1996.

Spear SL, et al. Surgery of the breast: principles and art. Lippincott-Raven; 1998.

Maillard GF, Montandon D, Goin J-L Plastic reconstructive breast surgery. Masson; 1983.

Lejour, M. Vertical mammaplasty and liposuction. Quality Medical; 1994.

Yalom M. A history of the breast. Ballantine; 1997.

Bamji A. Faces from the front. Gower Medical; 2017.

Meikle MC. Reconstructing faces – the art and wartime surgery of Gillies, Pickerill, McIndoe and Mowlem. Otago University Press; 2013.

Mayhew ER. The reconstruction of warriors – Archibald McIndoe, The Royal Airforce and the Guinea Pig Club. Frontline Books reprint 2010; 2004.

Regnault P, Daniel RK. Aesthetic plastic surgery. Little Brown; 1984.

Owsley JQ. Aesthetic facial surgery. W. B. Saunders; 1984.

Ho LCY, Klaassen MF, Mithraratne K. The congruent facelift: a 3D view. Springer; 2018.

Grabb WC, Smith JW. Plastic surgery. Little Brown; 1979.

Cormack GC, Lamberty GH. The arterial anatomy of skin flaps. Churchill Livingstone; 1986.

Barrett BM. Patient care in plastic surgery. Mosby; 1996.

Lüscher NJ Decubitus ulcers of the pelvic region: diagnosis and surgical therapy. Hogrefe & Huber; 1992.

Gruber RP, Peck GC. Rhinoplasty: state of the art. Mosby; 1993.

Appendix D: Time Frame for the FRACS (Plast) Exam

www.surgeons.org is an excellent resource, particularly under the category of education and training.

Candidates for the Final Fellowship Exam must have completed their training to the satisfaction of their surgical supervisors and be signed off to present for the final FRACS exam. There is an opening and closing date for registering as an exam candidate. The 2 written papers are sat in multiple standard venues throughout Australia and New Zealand.

5–6 weeks later the Clinical Vivas are held in designated locations. Results are not posted until both components have been completed and the Court of Examiners has met.

The final fellowship exams in plastic & reconstructive surgery for FRACS are held twice a year in either May/June or September/October.

Index

© Springer Nature Singapore Pte Ltd. 2018
M. F. Klaassen and E. Brown, *An Examiner's Guide to Professional
Plastic Surgery Exams*, https://doi.org/10.1007/978-981-13-0689-1

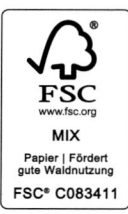

FSC
www.fsc.org

MIX

Papier | Fördert
gute Waldnutzung

FSC® C083411

Zeitfracht Medien GmbH
Ferdinand-Jühlke-Straße 7
99095 Erfurt, Deutschland
produktsicherheit@kolibri360.de